The
Politics
of **Stupid**

The
Politics

of **Stupid**

The Cure for Obesity

SUSAN POWTER

ATRIA BOOKS

New York   London   Toronto   Sydney

ATRIA BOOKS

A Division of Simon & Schuster, Inc.
1230 Avenue of the Americas
New York, NY 10020

First Atria Books trade paperback edition May 2008

ATRIA BOOKS and colophon are trademarks of Simon & Schuster, Inc.

For information about special discounts for bulk purchases,
please contact Simon & Schuster Special Sales at
1-800-456-6798 or business@simonandschuster.com.

Designed by Nancy Singer

Manufactured in the United States of America

10   9   8   7   6   5   4   3   2   1

Library of Congress Cataloging-in-Publication Data

Powter, Susan, date.
   The politics of stupid / Susan Powter.—1st Atria Books trade paperback ed.
     p. cm.
1. Women—Health and hygiene.   2. Physical fitness for women.
3. Women—Conduct of life.   4. Reducing diets.   5. Weight loss.   I. Title.

RA778.P88354 2008
613.2'5—dc22   2007049901

ISBN-13: 978-1-4165-8511-4
ISBN-10:   1-4165-8511-7

Here it is . . .

Sister . . .

We did it, my love . . .
We did it!

This book is dedicated to Amy

Contents

Foreword

The hardest thing about having a success is having a success. Oscar Wilde said something like it, except I'm sure he didn't use the word *success*. Oscar was talking about the hard part of getting what you want, and his language was certainly dressed in something much more nineteenth-century-sounding than the word *success*.

My generation's version of Oscar's thinking would be: once Leave It to Beaver, always Leave It to Beaver (who says quality is on the decline?), and the Beave and I, Susan Powter, have more in common than I ever dreamed possible.

I'm not sure what the Beave is doing now (or even if the Beave is still alive), so I can't honestly tell you what people expect from him, but I can promise you this: if I don't walk into an infomercial meeting screaming "Stop the Insanity" at the top of my lungs, the infomercial boys don't know what to do, and I'm thinking,

"The Beave has similar pressure simply because he is the Beave."

According to the marketing, creative, and writing wizards I'm up against in the infomercial world, "Stop the Insanity" was "the perfect formula." Overnight those three little words turned into one of the "most effective catchphrases in the weight-loss industry."

It's what they all wanted then, and it's what they are all still looking for now. The perfect sound bite. The one that sells, sells, sells.

And the only thing they want from me is?

"Yell it just once more, Susan . . ."

"Come on . . . Stop the . . . ? "

"How nutty is it?"

Insanity Two. Stop in the Name of Insanity, daughter of anything that resembles what I said way over ten years ago.

Rephrased: Go back and stay there, Susan. Don't move ahead. Stay right where the infomercial boys want you, now that they finally do understand it. Because don't forget (I never will), these are the same people who threw *Stop the Insanity* in the trash because it was too:

radical

loud

bald

aggressive

So I'll make one thing clear before I move forward: *Stop the Insanity* was a monster hit despite, or to spite (I certainly have it in me) them. They didn't get it, but *you* always did.

The only reason the corporate boys latched on was because of *you,* the women of America. It's you who heard "eat, breathe, and move" and "Norma Rae'd" it right into the spotlight. You were the ones who heard the weight-loss truth and jumped up with your signs held high, forcing the mills to grind to a stop.

It was *you,* not the wizards in the instant quick-fix-lying-through-their-teeth weight-loss-product-selling industry. You are the reason *Stop the Insanity* blew the roof off. Women. Millions of women got it in a big, big way.

Millions of women who were (and still are) looking for the strength and energy just to get through their/your day. Hundreds and thousands of Women trying to restore their bodies to some semblance of looking and feeling the way they want their bodies to look and feel. The boys in the how-to-sell-gadgets industries had nothing to do with *Stop the Insanity*. They don't own it, *you* do. Well, actually, I do.

The television-sell, market-research experts with their rhymes and reasons were dead wrong and scared to death, desperately afraid of you and me ever meeting, but according to the experts in the field of you and me, there was not much to worry about. There was no chance of that ever happening.

The women of America and Susan Powter, never! You

were never going to listen to, learn from, accept, watch on tele, or have anything to do with . . . me.

Just look at her, she's too . . . everything. They threw *Stop the Insanity* in the trash, literally, and got on with the quick fixes (that fix nothing) in the world of weight loss they do understand, the very profitable business of promising weight loss that never gets lost. It turns out that the experts in the field of you and me were wrong. *Stop the Insanity* was unstoppable. You and I did meet by the hundreds of thousands, and we continue to meet.

Of course, as soon as you did embrace *Stop the Insanity,* the experts in "what Women really want" jumped all over it and started advising me left, right, and center. If I wanted to "keep this thing going," I had to:

- Only talk weight loss in the most advertising-friendly, cute little sound bites.
- Say things that make the "average American housewife" (apparently, the only people who need to lose weight?) feel as if she was being respected. Operative words, feel as if? And, most important, I needed to:

> tone down
>
> soften up
>
> laugh a lot
>
> always be hap, hap, happy
>
> tell 'em (that would be you) what they want to hear

And never ever utter a political opinion.
"Women don't want to get tangled up in
politics."

True, these are quotes, folks, and I'd be glad to give
you the names and numbers of the men who said them.
They also said:

- Don't give them too much information.
- Keep it short and simple.

Because, I guess, all American women *are*? Listen, you
and I know that corporate America wouldn't know you
and me if we hit them over the head with you and me.

Turn on the television. Is your life anything close to
what is being advertised at you everywhere you turn? It
certainly isn't connected at all to mine or to the lives of
the thousands and thousands of Women I've met, the
Women I continue to meet every day, everywhere I go.

Who are these women walking around with a plastic spray bottle full of chemicals spraying their kids'
stuff, whistling while they work? What next, the white
knight riding in, resurrecting them from the dead? Snow
White ring a bell? A maid to seven midgets (or little
people) . . . political correctness aside, the woman was a
maid to seven little men and loved, loved, loved nothing
more than cleaning up after them. She died. Who are
these women?

These women are not me and they are not you. But it's
those moments blasted at us every second of every day

and now at warp speed that do affect/infect our lives. The powerful "atmospheric" suggestions about how your life should look, feel, and be; the standards that millions of women can't live up to. And when it comes to images created and directed at us by corporate America, there isn't a bigger, more damaging load of junk lurking around the parameters of your life than the weight-loss, wellness, fitness, standardized body image demanded of Women.

I never went into the infomercial business expecting high standards. In the thirty-minute late-night sellathon world, *integrity* and *honesty* were not words I expected to see at the top of any list. Don't ever forget just when it was that I walked into the late-night bullpen. Way before everyone and their mother thought they could do an infomercial and hit the jackpot. Back in the day when *Stop the Insanity* first appeared, the infomercial industry was still lighting cars on fire to prove the strength of the car wax they were begging you to buy. If you want trashy, I could (and will be glad to) tell you stories!

Then along comes *Stop the Insanity* . . . a beacon of light in a very dark world? No, simply a big, big hit despite the boys who think they know it all when it comes to what is going to make you pick up the phone and buy, buy, buy.

Do you want to know why *Stop the Insanity* was such a hit? It had nothing to do with any creative genius (excluding me, of course). There was not an expert in sight. It had nothing at all to do with anything anybody in the infomercial industry did, except plunk five cameras down during one of my live seminars. You know what they say about the timing necessary for most things to be enormously successful? Well, timing, did have something to do with *Stop the Insanity* being an enormous hit . . . the lack of time anyone spent on anything before they shot it.

They didn't believe in getting the simple truth about wellness to millions of Women, certainly not enough to spend an ounce of time on it. They didn't ask me what I was going to say, do, or wear. A five-camera shoot and nobody bothered to check what I was going to wear or say? Gone are the days . . . how lucky was I? Very lucky, I found out later as more and more people tried (consistently) to produce me out of me. I found out with a megahit that spawned six books, nine best-selling videos, and three infomercials just how lucky I'd been when *Stop the Insanity* first started. That infomercial was the last time I was allowed to do my work without intervention/interference, because nobody gave a crap. Everyone was too busy worrying about the suits to think about me.

Can you imagine the faces on the cash boys when I walked out onstage wearing those purple tights and a ripped sweatshirt? The first three rows, VIPs, looked like a wet-suit/shirt contest by the time I got to the ex-husband jokes.

"You can't talk about weight loss and your ex-husband in the same seminar. Oh God, what's she doing?"

"Don't joke with these women, act like an expert, stop with the funny. Weight loss is supposed to be serious!" "Jesus, she's flapping around a slice of bologna and calling it a pig's butt! Someone stop her!" But they couldn't.

A couple of thousand Women and I were completely

connected. We were laughing, learning, and loving the connection, and there was nothing the suits could do but attempt to fix it in the edit room, which they tried very hard to do. It was too late, I had already slipped in the one thing corporate America squashes the minute they hear it: an authentic voice with a twist . . . the truth.

Stop the Insanity

The only thing I did was tell the absolute truth about weight loss to a couple of thousand women, at the top of my lungs, without thinking about anything but the absolute truth about weight loss and how you could get as lean, as strong, and as healthy as you wanted. Blasphemy in the instant, quick-fix world of weight loss. *Vavoom:* it hit the air, you didn't surf past it. All of a sudden (I guess this is the "overnight" part of *overnight success* they keep referring to) along came the other product people with their offerings.

The Book

The literary community, the last vestige of civilization in the communications industry (according to their description of themselves) was light-years away from the sell, sell, sell world of the scummy infomercial boys. The literati came to the *Stop the Insanity* table with a very big offer— the first book—making it perfectly clear that "once ink is put to paper, it's immortal," which only means that more people than you ever wanted to know from are going to live forever. And the big question was: "Can she put this thing on paper?"

Everyone knows the infomercial world is bastardized beyond the point of no return. But ah, the book world! Aristocracy at its very best. Don't bother to pencil a parallel between these two worlds. Don't, for that matter, suggest that the two exist on the same planet because walking into a meeting with a room full of the literary elite is the polar opposite of meeting with the thirty-minute sellathon people. It's civilization versus third world. The air those literary folk breathe is different. Their oxygen is academic, mahogany-shelved, rich with description and, the gas that fills the lungs of the infomercial people smells like those bad cherry car air fresheners (which they'll gladly sell you for four easy payments of . . .) and never the two shall meet except when it comes to the sell.

The formula that works is the Krazy Glue that bonds the two together. The cash made from the big seller. The money generated, the volume sold, the mass production of it all. The catch-'em-and-sell-'em phrase that hits the list of the most sold items. The perfect formula.

As a literary/infomercial snowbird, calling both home when the season is right, I've seen it over and over again. You'd think six books in seven years would afford me some movement forward in the book biz, a world so full of creative people (again according to their gushing description of themselves), an inch or two perhaps? One look at the titles of my books *Stop the Insanity* and *Sober and Staying*

That Way: The Missing Link in the Cure for Alcoholism, the subjects alone suggest things have moved forward but, as true as true can be (and the Beave knows exactly how this feels), guess what was brilliantly suggested to me during the last "let's write another book" meeting?

How about another "Hey, Susan, wouldn't it be great if you wrote something just like . . ."

The same creative suggestion came from the video people, *lo mismo* from the TV and radio people . . . and I'm sure the Beave could back me up here, this stereotyping could have gone on forever unless you do what I did. Anyone who knows me for longer than a few seconds know exactly what's coming, but to ward (wasn't that the Beave's father's name?) off any confusion, let me tell you exactly what I did.

I am:

- ignoring everyone
- blowing them all off like bad habits
- covering my ears while they babble on . . .

Because I know and they don't. I am right, they are wrong. I know you want (and need) more than the old tried-and-true formulas that they keep handing you. I know you won't have any problem picking up the shovel and helping me throw dirt on *Stop the Insanity* of over ten years ago and move fast-forward to what's going on now.

I know for a fact that there is plenty of room in millions of Women's lives for all of the amazing life-changing information, motivation, and inspiration that you deserve to live in daily. Millions of people need these now, not when some creative genius in an office thinks they can handle it. When it comes to you solving the problems of "overfat" and "unfit" in your life, there is a whole lot you can do to change the way you look and feel forever.

The
Politics
of Stupid

one
Losing Weight

Losing weight is easy. You've lost weight over and over again. At least one of those diets worked for a couple of days/weeks at most, and . . . ?

You've lost weight . . . and gained it all back (and then some). According to the diet industry's own statistics, 98 percent of everybody who goes on a diet fails. Not good odds; not a table you would sit at in Vegas. Imagine a 98 percent chance that you are not going to win . . . would you throw your money down on that table? No, it wouldn't happen in Vegas, but it does happen with your body and your brain. The diet industry is a billion-dollar-a-year industry. Someone's buying what they are selling. Millions of people buying/believing that there is some system, formula, combination of foods, blood type, secret something that you still haven't found. But there isn't.

There isn't a diet on the planet Earth that works. I said it years ago—not one. If there were there wouldn't be a fat person on the planet. I would have found it, you would have found it, a whole lot of women (the primary victims of the diet industry) would have found it. Nobody would be fat if there were a diet that worked because we would all simply do what works and get on with it. The industry's own stats make the insanity of dieting very clear: 98 percent of everyone who goes on a diet (that would be *all* diets) fail.

But millions do. A billion dollars a year's worth of dieting. One of the truly insane insanities I was talking about when I said "Stop the Insanity" is dieting. Dieting to lose weight is actually the very definition of the word *insanity*. Doing the same thing over and over again and expecting different results. A billion-dollar-a-year industry says that a whole lot of people are (continually) dieting—that is to say, treating the symptoms and never solving the problems of overfat and unfit. Not a good way to do anything if solution is what you want. And if it's weight you want/need to lose, you *can*. Lose it and never find it again. Otherwise known as lose it forever, a permanent solution to overfat and unfit . . . there is such a thing and it's not achieved by dieting, obviously.

It's more than possible to solve the problems of overfat and unfit. It's common bloody sense. And solving the problems of overfat and unfit is also one of the most politically radical things any human body can do. "The most

revolutionary thing anybody can do is internal wellness,"
by Susan Powter.

I say it because:

A. It's true.
B. I did it.

I lost over 133 pounds and I have never found it again.
I look better and feel better at fifty than I did at twenty.
It's true. Life isn't going anywhere (until it does) and waking up every day with a foundation of wellness to live
from/in/with makes all the difference in everything. Life
is easier when you're not schlepping around a ton of fat,
when you have an ounce of energy to do the million
things you do every day. I'm still doing it all . . . every
woman I know is doing it all. What, has your life slowed
down? Do you have the luxury of time? Three kids and a
life later? Are you kidding? Life goes on, and when . . .

the back goes out, and it does . . .

the dental work needs doing, and it just did . . . surgery, thank you!

the broken bones of the past (and there are a few)
ache on a cold, rainy day, and they do . . .

. . . it's crap loads easier being lean, strong, healthy,
and a size two . . . argue with that. You can't. Nobody
would. I've asked the question thousands and thousands

of times (every seminar for how many years?). "If you could just wrinkle your nose . . . (à la *Bewitched*) and be lean, strong, healthy, and well, would you do so, or would you say "no, thank you." No need, I love the _____ (fill in the blank) pounds overweight I'm living with, I'd like to keep it." I've never gotten a "No, thank you, I love my stomach hanging halfway down my thighs, wouldn't trade it in for anything." I haven't heard it and I'm never going to hear it except for the sake of argument (what the delete button is designed for) because nobody telling the truth would say no to living in a body that is well, healthy, lean, and strong. Wellness works. Good food works. Movement works. Oxygen works. Thinking works.

Wellness revolutionized ("izes," it's current) my life and it will revolutionize yours. All of it absolutely true . . . so why can't I say there is a permanent solution to losing as much weight as you want to lose, increasing as much strength and energy as you want to increase, and loving the way you look and the way you feel . . . forever? Because it's not allowed. The lawyers want something more banal than permanent. Standards and practices will stop you in a heartbeat from uttering such a claim, even though what they do allow is stunning. No TV-segment producer is even going to understand what I'm talking about . . . for starters, they are all under twenty-one—everyone in TV *is* now, it's frightening . . . but the point is, it's not allowed. It's not allowed because once the simple truth is out, industries (a whole lot of them) will collapse. The Politics of Stupid is what's holding up more than you may have ever imagined possible, and understanding it has everything to do with the way you look and feel.

The minute you find out—or by the end of this book—how simple weight loss is, you'll have to take a moment, not an easy one, and admit you've been acting stupid. You are not stupid (or perhaps you are, but millions aren't), however; you absolutely have been *acting* stupid. Stupid as hell day after day after day for . . . years? Millions losing their lives, their health, their energy, their looks . . . go to an amusement park on any sunny day in any part of the country . . . some geographical regions are much worse than others . . . but have a look. I've met the smartest women—I'm talking brilliant—who don't have a clue. They've got no clue what to do. "How do I start? How, oh how, do I lose this weight?" I hear it a hundred times a day. It's stunning and real. There are a lot of reasons why you, women, are getting the megablasts in the war against an educated consumer . . . and believe me, you are—but before that dot is connected there is another vital connection that must be made, consider it the infrastructure for of your lean, strong, healthy life. Understanding the politics behind what has (when you think about it) made you do some stupid shit to your body is vital. Like you don't know preserved, spongy cakes with fake, fluorescent-white cream in the middle isn't food? Spending years searching for the time in your life for your life? Having no clue how to get rid of the fat that is hanging from all over your body?

You making the political connections directly connected to how you look and feel every day has everything to do with you re-gaining your body, your brain, and a whole lot more. The politics of a lifestyle that isn't working for millions of people is as real as it gets. The politics of the incorrect expert advice being doled out to you, and your family, is real. Billions of dollars spent on advertising, glamorizing, and "socializing" a lifestyle that isn't working for millions of people is real, and it works—the advertising, that is. The question is not "Why can't I (I stopped asking permission a long time ago) say there is a permanent solution to obesity?," the question is "Why aren't you hearing this simple, life-changing information, these absolute facts, everywhere you turn?" Being completely clear about the Politics of Stupid is the answer if you are:

fat

unfit

exhausted

diseased

hate the way you look and feel

desperately want to feel well

Any/all of the above is/are what the Politics of Stupid is about. Making this connection is as vital to weight loss as eat, breathe, move, and think is and, it all is. You are, certainly, not alone.

Obesity is epidemic. An epidemic. Millions of people

suffering from the exact same thing? What? Suffering from what? Look, up in the sky, it's a gene, it's a virus, it's a . . . *Lifestyle*. It's a lifestyle "issue." A lifestyle that is affecting/infecting millions of people.

Epidemic numbers of people don't have a clue about what to put into their mouths. Millions of people with the same willpower "issues"? Millions of people suffering from the same "inner-child trauma"? Hundreds of thousands of weakhearted people? It's getting harder, by the second, to blame it on childhood trauma, genes, your mother being a horror, because the facts are:

- America is second in the world in heart disease.
- Obesity is epidemic.
- Childhood obesity has increased 54 percent in the last fifteen years.
- Cancers are epidemic.

All of the above are lifestyle matters or diseases, and lifestyle can (easily) be changed forever. Which changes the way you look and feel forever. Nothing complicated about that.

Wellness changed my life . . . in more ways than I ever dreamed possible, I mean that literally . . . and it will change yours. To be physically free from exhaustion is freedom. Having the lean muscle mass (metabolically the most active tissue in the human body) to stand, sit, bend, pick up, run around after . . . all the things you are doing now without the strength and energy to do them . . . is freedom. Activating your heart/lung systems, the oxygen-processing center of your body, is freedom. Igniting your metabolic rate and burning as much fat as you want to burn is freedom. And freedom is political.

Millions of people are dying (literally) for the information, inspiration, and motivation to get physically well enough to get through a day. There's no question that it's time to move forward. It's way past time that you got on with living your life in energy and strength in a lean, strong, beautiful, well body. And there's only one way on earth to do it.

You've got to eat.
You've got to breathe,
You've got to move. And . . .
You've got to think.

Eat, breathe, move, and think are solutions for the problems of overfat and unfit. Your understanding the politics of a lifestyle that affects/infects you and your family, daily, and knowing how to avoid it like the plague that it is, is a permanent solution. There's no question that politics has to be a part of any/all discussions connected to getting lean, strong, healthy, and well, and certainly is (i.e., the title) but, most important and quite simple, is you having everything you need to change what isn't working in your life. "I've been fat and I've been fit, fit is better," and it is.

Movement Forward

It may be way past time that you took care of this "little weight problem" of yours, but it's never too late. And, O mighty female consumer, you are exactly the person who's going to change . . . well, everything, but for now, it's all about your body. There has been a massive change in consumer consciousness in the land while I've been girding the last loin of my loins for battle. I've watched it happen. It's all about Women.

Women stronger at forty than we were at twenty. Hundreds and thousands of women over forty having babies, never before in history, a massive "cultural" change that ripples out beyond our wildest dreams. Menopause couldn't be mentioned just one generation ago; not something my mother was allowed to mention . . . certainly not the surgically induced menopause she barely made it through. Well, one generation later, *this* menopausal mother—and I am one—and millions of other mothers are making very, very different decisions about:

the foods they eat

the healing they are choosing

the medicines they are not choosing anymore and why they're not choosing them.

Professions are being changed, forever, by what we are, and are no longer, accepting. Women are pirating back what is and always was ours; everything from physical strength and energy to birth, healing, our bodies, our brains, our voices. And one hell of a good place to start reclaiming more than you may have ever imagined possible is wellness, which is now included under a much bigger umbrella than just weight loss, and is the only way weight gets lost. Internally activating or, as I like to think of it, resurrection from the walking dead millions are "waking up" in daily. That's where I come in, and getting more obvious by the second, that's where the politics of it all comes in and, it does.

There's a whole lot more available today—when it comes to you reclaiming your body, your brain, and your life—than there was back in the day. *Holistic* mean anything to anybody? Naturopathy, homeopathy, craniopathy, herbs, alternative, Mother Nature and all her gifts . . . these are not such freaky ideas anymore. And the reason is that a very powerful consumer market demanded alternatives to what had been happening for far too long. You, mother, tired of the same old, same old prescription for the same old, same old ear infection, given to you by the same old, same old pediatrician. Mothers intuitively questioning so-called experts about such things as autism, vaccinations, baby formulas—not just the junk the doctors insisted, for years, was far more convenient and better for baby than breast-feeding, the tried-and-true formulas that we no longer believe in. Alternative . . . to what? Mention St.-John's-wort back in the day, people thought I was talking about a skin condition. Suggest ginkgo ten years ago and you could pretty much expect to be accused of witchcraft. Homeopathy, until very recently, was thought to be a sexual preference, but not anymore.

Your solving the problems of overfat and unfit in your life has everything to do with you dusting off the "tiara" and acting like the powerful consumer you are and being very clear about how politically powerful you are every time you walk down the aisles of your grocery store. It's true . . . you don't have to go any farther than your local grocery store to know exactly what I'm talking about. Food is connected to how you look and feel . . . you'd agree with that because nobody wouldn't at this point. Yes, what you put into your mouth, into your body, has everything to do with how you look and feel on the out-side. The Zen of food is simple. I'll give you a few bumper stickers.

Junk in, junk out.

Eat dough, look like dough.

Eat shit, look and feel like shit.

By, Susan Powter.

Food is directly connected to the top four killers in the United States and directly connected to obesity . . . there is no question about that anymore. And the food industry is a big one. A $276-billion-dollar-a-year in-dustry . . . that's a *very* big one. And here's an absolute fact about the all-American lifestyle that explains much: 85 percent of the consumer market for the $276-billion-dollar food industry is . . . ? Who's doing the grocery shopping in your house. No need to send me an e-mail if you are one of the (*very* few) men doing the weekly grocery shopping; I'm not interested and I'm not talking about you. I'm talking to the majority (in more ways than one) walking the aisles week after week after week for years.

Women.

Queens of the aisles, you are. Millions of Women roaming the aisles of the grocery stores have everything to do with a whole lot of very political issues, and certainly everything to do with obesity. And it's not coincidental that Women are also the primary victims of the diet industry. A couple of ways to control the masses are:

- starvation, otherwise known as dieting—it works brilliantly
- poison them . . . they will be too tired and toxic to
- confuse the hell out of them, completely and absolutely, about the most basic things like what to put into their mouth.

Spin them in circles so they spend all their energy on "vital" questions like "carbs vs. protein?" The truth is that you, the most powerful consumer market in the country today, are too tired, toxic, overfat, and unfit to even think about _____ (fill in the blank). Buried alive in your own life even though everywhere you turn "convenient," "value," "bargain," "instant," "easy," "the very best for you and your family," "all for the low, low price of" is being blasted at you at the speed of light. Maybe you haven't been able to put your finger on exactly what it is, but you've known for a long time that something is wrong. Terribly wrong . . . and you really don't have a clue about what to do, or where to start. And it's not because you are stupid. The *stupid* in the title of this book doesn't imply that you are. Millions of women are not stupid, but stupid millions of women are acting.

You are overworked, underpaid (not paid at all), buried alive in your life, overfat, unfit, exhausted, and acting stupid. So, yep . . . it works. Numb them and dumb them and they'll be numbed and dumbed. Heavily funded campaigns ("campaigns"—note the wording, ladies, the wording) designed to sell you, and they work. Your life and its style, or lack of it, is directly connected to the way you look and feel and to thousands of symptoms that millions don't have to suffer from. Lifestyle is the connection. Lifestyle, and looking and feeling like hell, are directly connected no matter how many millions of dollars are spent trying to convince you otherwise. Eighty-five percent of all diseases can be directly attributed to lifestyle. The organization that says this, the American Medical Association, is not acting as if lifestyle could (and it can) fix 85 percent of the problems millions of people are suffering from, are they? Not at all.

This book and everything I'm doing now is based on an idea I had years ago. The concept of exchanging stuff that you made a mistake in buying. Yeah, if you don't like it you exchange it, don't you? I've seen women drive bloody miles to exchange a piece of clothing that, once home, was wrong. You spend money on it and it doesn't work, you exchange it. You'd sure as hell exchange anything if it affected every waking moment of your life. If it could literally save your life, and it can, would you exchange what you are doing right now for it? There's no chance you would just "oh well" it to the grave; no way. That would be stupid. Exactly. But millions are doing just that when it comes to the most important of important, the one thing all the other stuff is based on, because without your health, you ain't got nothing by, Me.

My mother died at fifty-two. Money in the bank, a Jaguar in the garage, everything most people want . . . and it was lifestyle that killed her. A 1950s housewife, never knew anyone but the man she was married to for thirty-three years (don't start glorifying that number; it was hell), she listened to everything her doctor, priest, and husband said. Ate like they told her. Lived like they told her. Had all the surgeries they told her to have. Never questioned any of them, well . . .

Well, well, well, a whole lot has changed just one generation later, and the very least of it is the difference between what my mother and I eat, breathe, move, and think. Now I'm fifty years old, and lifestyle's got a much harder job of killing me than it did her. It wouldn't have been considered ladylike if my mother did the yoga pelvic moves I did this morning . . . take it from there. The point is, if you look in the mirror today and don't like what you see, if you don't like the end results of the lifestyle you are living, you can change it. My mother didn't have a choice. We do.

Exchange the lifestyle you are living, which in my brain turned into an obvious yet brilliant weight-loss program. A lifestyle X-change program that quite simply (and it all is) means you are going to X-change one lifestyle habit at a time, and very soon, before you know it you've X-changed the lifestyle that doesn't work for you . . . for the millions of you.

Change is what you are about to do. Change what you are putting in and you will change what is on the outside. Change inactive for active and you change much, much more than just burning fat. Change weak for strong, tired for energized . . . I can and will go on, but for now let's stick with the conception of your program by, me. What happened in my brain was a lifestyle "X-change" program.

X-change a lifestyle that isn't working for a style of life that does. Sometimes as corny as it is, it has to be. X-ing out what isn't working for what does work is the bottom-line truth of weight loss . . . and literally what you are going to do. That's what the Politics of Stupid is . . . you understanding that if millions are doing the same wrong thing, their mistake must be based on something more than you not being able to "figure it out." Connecting the dots and the only way on the planet Earth to lose weight. A weight-loss program that takes everything to a new level by using everything available in this day and age to "every-body" who wants it.

The Internet changed everything for me. Very little will ever come between me and "every-body" who wants to be well again. Private training will never be the same . . . and it's about time. I've watched, waited, and worked very hard for the last fifteen years in order to be exactly where I am right now. "Direct" from me to you is the only way to go, and now we can. The book you are holding in your hands, my face, my voice, my life on www.susanpowteronline.com . . . these are "directly" connected to you losing as much weight as you want to lose via space. There was no chance in hell any of this could have happened just five short years ago. But the biz of getting the simple truth about wellness and life-changing information to you is far more complicated than most will ever understand unless you've been an infomercial queen or king.

Who is Ron Popeel? The "king" to my "queen," you could say. Back in the day, you couldn't imagine what it took to get the truth out. Me sandwiched between publishers, video houses, syndicators, lawyers, agents, production horror everywhere I turned. To hell with artistic integrity . . . that's not why I left; it was just impossible to get anything done properly, honestly, and without getting screwed to the wall, and I was.

Here are the facts. I do wellness. I do it every day: eat, breathe, move, and think. Translating that life-changing information to you (all the millions of you) should be simple, and, at long last, it is. For the first time in history, you can, and will essentially, come live with me. That's what we are going to be doing. Reality . . . actual reality. Bowing to the Queen of Everything, Madonna, what I'm saying is beyond Truth or Dare. It would have happened earlier, but the "experts" wouldn't listen to me, so I kept going and going and going until someone did. Now that the mediums (all of them) of communication have changed so dramatically and the TV networks (all of them) have lost their monopoly, it's possible. Since those young Internet pranksters that the stiff white corporate boys laughed at just a few short years ago have taken over the world, you and I have much much more opportunity. This program is one of the biggest things that got me off the farm and back into the world . . . I'm talking about your lifestyle X-change program, delivered to your life via book, audios, videos, and by me, "directly" transported into your life via www.susanpowteronline.com! Retirement over . . . she's back, folks.

Never before has getting vitally important information been so easy, and never before has it been more important. Oh, it's global, people, and it's political. As a matter of absolute fact, wellness is the only hope this planet has of surviving, by, Susan Powter. Becoming a thinking consumer. An educated consumer. Awareness abounding. Internal wellness . . . you getting your body lean, strong, healthy, and well . . . this is as green as it gets, and it's about damn time the connection was made. I'm beginning to resent being shoved off to the side of all the green discussions as simply a fitness expert. First, the word *expert* offends the hell out of me, and second, there isn't anything more green "any-body" can do than wellness.

Imagine how pissed all the experts of the past would be at the idea of Women sharing the truth . . . our experiences, our expertise, and changing how we live. "I'm just a housewife who figured it out and started talking to other housewives" . . . that is exactly what *Stop the Insanity* was about and always will be about. Women, networking and connecting the dots to the truth when they hear it, and now we can do it globally with far fewer anythings in between me and you. The program is simple. Take back what you don't like and are no longer going to live with. X-change a lifestyle, one life-changing habit at a time, that isn't working, and before you know it (literally), you have changed everything. Change a choice, change your life—this is real . . . your body and your brain are directly connected, Dr. Dr. The way to change is by creating a style of life that fits you, that gets you the end results you want . . . a daily life that works for you and your family. Overfat doesn't suit you. Lean will. Unfit doesn't work. Fit does. Unwell doesn't look or feel good. This lifestyle X-change program will revolutionize your life. I've waited years to say that because it's the only way to do it and it's the truth.

two

Reclaiming the Throne

I've come back to work for a couple of reasons. After having fired everyone (a whole lot in that one infamous paragraph) and started the finale of my child-rearing years, I'm exactly where I want to be and have worked very hard to be. And the technology I've waited for years to catch up to me is right where I want it to be. None more important (certainly for weight loss) than the Internet. One of the most astounding cultural changes any of us will ever witness in our lifetime (unless you were around at the beginning of industrialization . . . and oh, what a success that's been), the Web is now my infrastructure for revolutionizing weight loss. Exactly what I intend to do and one of the only things powerful enough to get me to dust off the throne . . .

It's all in place. Everything is in the perfect place to

help millions of people all over the world get lean, strong, and healthy. And I intend to take full advantage of this powerful window of opportunity. One of the very annoying things about me is that "it" doesn't change. As my twenty-five-year-old son made clear to me years ago, "There is no low to this high." In other words, every body needs me. Fitness is for everyone. Wellness is the greatest common denominator. Your gender, race, religion, or politics don't matter. That's right. None of it matters because if you are human, if you live in a human body, then what I'm saying applies to you. It doesn't matter what you think of me, what I'm saying applies.

"Where has she been?" I'll answer that question before it's asked. I left and went to live on a horse farm with my baby because I was heartsick. For every ten people who claimed that *Stop the Insanity* was their own, the fact is, it was, and is, mine. I wrote every word. I did every seminar. I had very very little help doing all the work that those three words conjured for a whole lot of people.

Something that happened one morning, just before the letter, explains much. Sitting in front of the palatial home of my manager, I realized that I was funding all of it. Lifestyles I wasn't living, funded by me. Without me, they couldn't live them, and they haven't since. None of them. The problem with claiming the success of Susan Powter or *Stop the Insanity* is doing it again . . . Make it "happen" again. They haven't. A whole lot of people have realized in the last ten years that to do Susan Powter you need Susan Powter. I had to get that message across before I did it again. To spite, I told you I had it in me, despite everyone who believed *they* did it for me.

Cut off my nose to spite my face or a point that had to be made before I went out and did it again. If you think I'm all about love and acceptance, then you don't even know whose book you are reading because I'm not. Not at all. It's the other side of loving I'm talking about. The side never spoken about, even though you can't have love without it. Always what's unsaid because it's not allowed. Fury. A vital passion in every healthy persons life, unless you don't see a thing that's happening all around you? Unless you are dead, you have to be bloody furious. I hate like poison and I hate forever. I'll take it to the grave with me and everyone will know it. I've got quite a story to tell—the last four years alone, and you know I will be telling it, but I want to talk about building the infrastructure so that every human body on earth can get lean, strong, and healthy. So let's get back to that horse farm and my baby. You could only imagine my surprise when I looked up from the diaper pail and heard the words *high-protein weight loss*. Impossible.

High Protein

My first thought when I heard the name "Atkins" was, "Didn't someone shoot that guy?" No, that was the Scarsdale Diet guy, selling the same huge protein weight-loss lie. What's been going on in the weight-loss (that never stays lost) business while I was off not going insane . . . well, it's insane. High-protein masters cleansing you left, right, and center, rerouting intestines, stomachs being tied, just a few examples of the same-old same old. *Stop the Insanity* all over again, only now more than ever.

For God's sake, high protein? Haven't you already done that? You have . . . in the seventies. Back in the day, you separated the burger from the bun and only ate the burger, but that was way before thirty-five years of grassroots education. Today, there is no way "any-body" can eat the foods the high-protein boys are telling them to eat and not include the top five killers (heart disease, stroke, hypertension, obseity, cancer) in the United States because these killers are directly connected to high-protein eating.

High protein for weight loss, the goal being ketosis? Wrong. Who knew back then, but you know now. Saturated fat, cholesterol, poisons, hormones, horrifying manufacturing conditions . . . there is nothing new about any of it. Feces-covered meat. You've seen it. Streamlined inspection systems that inspect nothing. *E. coli* everywhere . . . it was in this morning's news—again. What (about all of it) doesn't affect your health? Political, oh without a doubt, but still not what got me up and out. What pissed me off enough to come back to work was how many people, women primarily, fell for the high-protein weight-loss lie . . . again. I couldn't believe it. Not for a second did I think the high-protein load of bull could become the megahit it became, but somehow *it did*. And so I came back to work to stalk Atkins. Not just any diet lie could pull me out of seclusion . . . only the resurrection of something as ridiculous as the high-protein weight-loss cant from the seventies could do it. My only motivation in hanging out the shingle again was Atkins . . . and then he died.

Eating the most infected, gross, high-fat, cholesterol-ridden, putrid foods in our food system doesn't work on many, many levels. Eating high-protein foods to solve the (epidemic) problem of obesity is insane.

You've never heard and you won't ever hear anybody say, "Oh my God, my doctor just told me my arteries are ninety percent occluded, and it's because I'm suffering from a protein deficiency."

There's no chance in hell you will ever hear anybody say, "I just got off the scale and I'm tipping three hundred pounds. Apparently I've got a protein deficiency?"

Nor will you ever hear, "My aunt just died from a stroke, and if only we'd known about her protein deficiency, we could have saved her."

You'll never hear these words because too little protein is not the problem. As a matter of (absolute) fact, way too much protein has everything to do with occluded arteries, obesity, and stroke, but for now let's stick with weight loss. Ah, the politics of the high-protein weight-loss lie. Making this simple political connection is as easy as it gets . . . let's start by looking at the lobbies, shall we? The meat and dairy boys . . . any question about how much control they've had for how long? Any idea how heavily they fund (having the last word) almost everything? Things like:

- your children's education; have a look you'll see
- your "health care" systems, totally and absolutely
- the media . . .

If it's well-funded campaigns you are interested in, you might want to look into these two enormously powerful groups—the meat lobby and the dairy lobby—that have for years had total control of more than you may have ever thought affects how you live. You gotta love the Internet, but not if you don't want to be exposed to some ugly truths. It's not difficult today to see that most of what we've all been told is good for us . . . isn't. The pillars of the past have crumbled under their own lies. Health statistics speak volumes about the experts who have been in charge of health for years.

Food pyramids . . . wrong! Government-approved (and funded) meat and milk for the majority . . . grains for the heathens. Health freaks . . . blasphemy! Theories about the connection between what you eat and such mysterious things as heart disease. The lobbies fought the truth every step of the way until very, very recently. Their own statistics put them in the grave, and the foods they've been telling people to eat have put millions in the grave. Oh, how they fought.

Their products connected to heart disease! Nonsense. For years, any organization that tried to expose this truth was squashed. What is happening today with food is something you've seen happen before. Another industry lying and hiding the truth for years. Killing millions. Normalizing, glamorizing, and advertising their wares when they knew what was really going on for over forty years. I'm talking about the tobacco industry. The food industry is not much different. Affecting millions biochemically. Creating disease absolutely. Making millions sick, all the while funding study after study to prove those pesky consumer advocates insane! There is very little chance you haven't made the direct connection between your food supply and the old Norman Rockwell meat-and-potato thinking of the past no longer existing.

Branding is real. My mother was "branded," her mother was . . . but you and I don't have to be. We don't have to be exposed. Hot iron to the flesh is what branding is about, and it works. Everything changes when millions put together the pieces of the puzzles that affect us all. And these "annoying women" sharing what they know . . . they're changing everything. Not much pisses the "deans" of the "institutions" off more. The high-protein weight-loss resurrection is one of the most astounding things I've ever seen. "Carbs vs. protein" is again the language of weight loss. Industry after industry was built on it. Splenda was birthed from it! And the politics of pulling this particular wool (an insult to sheep) over the eyes of millions of women is stunning.

A. It had already been done, over thirty-five years ago, and if it had worked then, epidemic levels obesity wouldn't be a fact of life now.

Atkins died, but, unfortunately, his old and tired (two of the things his diet will make you) high protein didn't.

The high-protein boys continued to use a dead doctor as a mascot for a couple of strong sell, sell, sell-'em years and have only recently lost their grip on the brains of the masses . . . because it doesn't work, and people feel (and look) like shit when they're on it. It's mortifying, and deadly. And it was enough to get me off the horse farm. I'm back, and whether you are thrilled that I am or wish I'd stayed on the farm . . . either way, you can put the blame on Atkins.

Atkins and gastric bypass were two very good reasons for me to come back to work and say again what I said over a decade ago and kept on saying for a decade. The nineties weren't that long ago, but a lifetime ago compared to the world we live in today. I've watched the world change. Every industry I've been involved in—books, audios, videos, manufacturing, distribution—has changed forever. The business of getting vitally important information to millions of people has also changed forever and completely, and I'm thrilled. If you want to lose weight, you have to change your lifestyle. You need to eat whole real foods vs. processed junk; you need activity vs. inactivity; you need lean muscle mass and strength not weakness; you need cardio endurance; energy vs. exhaustion; you need well not unwell.

It's not easy being me. I go as far back as Fen-phen and Redux . . . remember? It wasn't that long ago that these two government-approved, handed-out-like-candy, little weight-loss helpers were being scarfed down by millions of women. Then, oops, heart problems along with a holy host of other side effects. I was in a boardroom (very, very bored) with some of the corporate boys who began the Fen-phen craze, and was told, "It costs us pennies to hand them a pill vs. a few dollars to run them through a healthy regimen . . . we can make millions with the pill." Diet pills always and forever. That never changes, and if you don't think pharmacology is political, then you haven't seen or read anything in years. Diet pills . . . the names have been changed to protect . . . *there's* a saying that needs no ending and applies. The names mean very little. You looking for the pill that will fix this obesity thing, is simply nuts. Diet pills . . . I did them. At 260 pounds, I took the pills my doctor gave me and I lost weight. A bunch of it really fast . . . and gained it all back and then some. Of course I lost weight when I did speed, but can anyone really prescribe diet pills as a solution for overfat and unfit? Taking a pill to lose weight has nothing to do with wellness and never has or ever will solve the problems of overfat or unfit. Just another billion-dollar—*several*-billion-dollar—industry that has yet to do what they continually say they will do.

Today, there are more weight-loss-pill promises than it's worth keeping track of, which says everything that needs saying about how effective the never-ending promise of diet pills is. However, all the pill promises in the world don't come close to winning "The Most Insane Weight-Loss Solution-from-the-Experts" Award. Diet pills were not enough to pull me out of exile . . . no, no. Hands down, the winners were gastric bypass surgery and high protein.

Gastric Bypass

Hmm, what to say about this new and improved expert (only the most expert can administer it, those certified by the AMA) procedure given to fat people. Reroute your intestines. Surgically induce extreme dieting. That'll solve the problem. Stunningly wrong, unabashed in the chutzpah it takes to sell this absurdity, and oh, how they are sell, sell, selling people on the surgical solution for fat. Lean, strong, and healthy has nothing to do with "creating a small gastric pouch from the patient's original stomach then dividing the jejunum, the second segment of the small bowel, and connecting it to the gastric pouch, then reconnecting the bowel to the segment of small bowel that is connected to the gastric pouch." And just a few of the side effects are . . . ?

lung problems, pneumonia, blood clots

infection

death

bleeding

bowel blockage

leakage of bowel content into abdomen

chronic nutritional problems; protein, vitamin, and mineral deficiencies

stomach-outlet blockage

less-than-desired weight loss

more-than-desired weight loss

returned fertility leading to unplanned pregnancy

possible birth defects related to vitamin and mineral deficiencies of mother

nausea, vomiting, temporary hair loss, food intolerances, changed bowel habits, loss of muscle mass . . .

Even if you have the surgery—and so many have—you still have to change your lifestyle . . . the very thing that got you fat in the first place . . . and a much better place to solve the problems of overfat and unfit than an operating table. Reread this last sentence; it makes perfect sense. Actually, nothing more needs to be said about gastric bypass surgery than what is being said by the people who've had it. I hear from them daily and have spoken, many times, with the victims of this extraordinarily profitable procedure.

For example, Anne from Tennesse writes:

I need your help—I recently had gastric bypass surgery and am following my doctor's directions. When I drink hot or cold liquid, I get this excruciating pain across my stomach that doubles me over. I've also been getting very light-headed with just minimal physical activity, like standing up or walking up the steps. Do you have any answers for me?

Candace from Massachusetts writes:

Susan, you talk about brown rice as being very healthy for you, but once you've had gastric bypass surgery, it is pretty much a no-no. That along with pasta and bread because they take in liquid after they enter the stomach pouch, which can cause pain and swelling. Do you have any alternatives?

MaryKate from Oregon writes:

Susan, I recently lost a very good friend to what I call gastric bypass butchery. I know that you would never become a proponent of this [procedure], but could you please use your voice to put some information out there so people truly realize how dangerous it is. Did you know a study by researchers at the University of Washington found that one in fifty people dies within one month of having gastric bypass surgery, and that jumps nearly five fold if the surgeon is inexperienced. These are terrible statistics and everyone should know the facts!

It's not difficult to admit, in this day and age, that professional ethics have been skewed forever by the systems that rule them, and us. Lobbying mean anything to you? If it does, you must know that it applies to all industry. Gone are the days when the medical professions can be romanticized. If not, consider, your bubble broken. It has been horrifying for me watching this fog descend on thinking people. Surgery for this little weight-loss issue of yours, it is the suggestion pumped directly into brains, like oxygen in Vegas, it's real and brilliantly well funded by some mighty big boys. Surgery to solve the problem of obesity . . . let's see, how many industries involved in that culturally saturated nonthinking? Right off the bat, only three of many . . .

medical (the AMA)

insurance

pharmaceutical

And the hundreds of other industries that these three breed. No need to spend much more energy on determining just how insane a solution it's not. A far better way to spend your precious energy is to simply become aware of what is happening, naming it, the politics of a lifestyle that is absolutely affecting/infecting you daily, and getting on with changing it.

When it comes to getting the help of the surgical experts, bypass the bypass boys.

It'll only take a paragraph or two to explain how gastric bypass doesn't and can never, work. And, again, it's indisputable when you look at the facts of the weight-loss matter. If you live in a human body, you have to eat to be lean; once the bypass boys have rerouted you, you can't. You have to move to burn fat, and if you can only eat a few teaspoons of the same stuff you were eating to get fat, you've got a couple of problems. It's very, very hard to burn fat, build lean muscle mass, and activate your body internally when you are starving. Not only does the amount of calories you have to eat to get lean become a huge problem, but the kinds of fuel your body must have to be well . . . no can do. Gastric bypass makes looking and feeling good almost impossible. The people who've had it make that really clear.

Marilyn writes:

Susan, I'm writing to you out of desperation—I have lost 175 pounds after bypass surgery but I have skin hanging everywhere! My arms, my thighs, my tummy! Can you recommend any exercises to tighten this up?

Nancy writes:

Susan, I just saw you give a speech and you look amazing and you inspired me to write to you to ask for your help. I am struggling with the skin that is dripping off my body. I had lap-band surgery, and while I was successful in losing weight, my body looks HORRIBLE. I have so much loose skin I actually have to tuck it into my clothes. I can't afford plastic surgery and am sick of walking around like this. Can you help me?

Kayla writes:

I'm so depressed. I feel like I've been cheated. I bought in to all the promises of weight-loss surgery because I hated the way I looked. After struggling with major health problems after the surgery, I've finally got my body back to some type of "normal." The problem is the way my body looks now. Everything sags, everything droops, and everything hangs. It is so depressing. My breasts have what seems like sheets of extra skin, not to mention the rest of my body . . .

And don't forget to add enormous amounts of hanging skin to one of the most hideous side-effect lists I've ever seen. This is exactly what happens when you "lose weight" via starvation or dieting. Another human-body fact that even your doctor wouldn't be stupid enough to argue with is:

The Problem with Dieting

When you diet, taking in fewer calories than you expend, four things happen to the human (every human) body. The first thing that happens when you take in less than you expend is:

1. Your body walks around in a constant state of high-caloric craving. This is not an eating disorder. It's not about being "addicted" to food and not a willpower "issue." It's actually your body screaming at you to eat the cake, grab the fries, eat anything with calories—fuel. Shoving food into your mouth every afternoon and all evening is not the emotional issue the self-love experts like to say

it is. It's basic biology. Let's look at the biology, shall we?

The second thing that happens when you take in less than you expend is:

2. Your body metabolically slows down to whatever you are taking in, both in quantity and quality. Functioning like a slug?

The third thing that happens to the human body—yours—when you take in less than you expend is:

3. Your body burns lean muscle mass as fuel. Because you aren't putting enough fuel in, your body will use lean muscle as fuel.

And, my favorite little caloric fact—because it's just so telling and every woman who's dieted instinctively knows this and now you'll know why—is the fourth thing that happens to every human body when you take in less than you expend:

4. Your brilliant body will store the fuel that lasts the longest in famine. And that fuel is . . . ? Fat.

Diets make you fatter and weaker; you know that. And diets don't work; you also know that. Gastric bypass surgery is a surgically imposed *diet*. Which means, it doesn't work.

These four basic facts (and they are) of the human body change much when you think about them. Four basic truths about the human body that beg the question "How much fuel/food do you need if not eating enough (dieting) and eating total crap affects whether or not you lose weight?"

And the answer is found in a blast from the past, namely, the old daily caloric consumption chart. This chart is more applicable now than ever and an oak in the infrastructure of you solving this little weight-loss problem of yours once and for all. The truth never changes, and now it's here for all to see.

Directly from the American Medical Association, an absolute fact of the weight-loss matter that, again, interestingly enough, isn't spoken about, certainly not as much as carbs vs. protein.

As you can see, how much fuel you need depends on a couple of things, specifically how much you weigh and how active you are. Logically. If it's fat you want to lose, then you must eat, and unless you sit around all day doing nothing, (not a description of any Woman's day I know of), then you need quite a bit of fuel to get through a day.

When you're taking in less than you expend—otherwise known as every diet I've ever heard of—how many times have you heard "eat a couple of thousand calories a day, minimum, and make sure it's the highest-quality food"? Only once would be the answer, because if you did (when you do) you would look and feel fabulous . . . problem solved. But for the sake of infrastructure staging (and we are), let's go over Caloric Consumption 101.

Daily Caloric Consumption Predictions for Women

Resting calories (doing nothing)
Low activity (low-impact walking, cycling 2–3 times a week)
Medium activity (low-impact walking or cycling 4–5 times a week)
High activity (low-impact walking or cycling 6–7 times a week)

Your Weight (Pounds)	Resting Calories	Low Activity	Medium Activity	High Activity
100	**1,120**	**1,450**	**1,570**	**1,680**
110	1,150	1,490	1,600	1,720
120	1,190	1,550	1,670	1,780
130	1,220	1,580	1,700	1,830
140	1,250	1,630	1,750	1,880
150	**1,280**	**1,660**	**1,800**	**1,920**
160	1,320	1,720	1,850	1,980
170	1,350	1,750	1,890	2,000
180	1,380	1,790	1,930	2,070
190	1,420	1,850	1,990	2,100
200	**1,450**	**1,880**	**2,030**	**2,180**
210	1,480	1,950	2,050	2,200
220	1,513	1,970	2,100	2,270
230	1,540	2,000	2,160	2,300
240	1,580	2,050	2,200	2,400
250	**1,610**	**2,090**	**2,250**	**2,410**
260	1,640	2,130	2,300	2,460
270	1,676	2,170	2,350	2,500
280	1,710	2,220	2,400	2,560
290	1,740	2,260	2,440	2,600
300	**1,770**	**2,480**	**2,500**	**2,660**

Sources:
Mayo Clinic Report, *volume 163 (1998);* American Journal of Clinical Nutrition, *volume 44 (1986), 1–19.*

Daily Caloric Consumption

You need lots of fuel every day if you do anything. Starting with three squares, no exception, at the very least. If it's body fat you want to burn (and you do), you must eat. If it's body fat you want to lose (and it is), you must move. If you are not doing those two things and are losing weight, especially what's considered a winning weight loss or a biggest loser number, you are not burning body fat. Ten, twenty, thirty pounds in one week! There are lawyers, doctors, and trainers surrounding a TV show that big (pardon the pun) and still, absolutely wrong. A thirty-pound weight loss in one week, wrong. The four human-body facts (reread them) that happen when you take in less than you expend are absolute so, those numbers are not about fat loss. Those successful weight-loss numbers are mostly water and lean muscle mass, because (another annoying biological fact) an absolute fact of the human (all) body matter is:

The human body can process only two pounds of fat a week. Meaning, if you lose more than two pounds a week, what you are losing above that number is water and lean muscle . . . unless, of course, you:

A. Are a genetic mutant
B. Don't live in a human body

If you want to solve the problem of overfat forever, two things you really don't want to lose are water (because the minute you drink some, you gain it back) and lean muscle (because metabolically it's the most active tissue in the human body, all humans' bodies). Losing the most active tissue in the human body means you are:

A. Losing the wrong thing
B. Really not going to have the strength you need to get through the day

And it also means your body is doing what all human bodies do when they lose impossible amounts of "weight" in stupid amounts of time via starvation. It means your body is storing the fuel that lasts the longest in famine . . . fat.

All of which will be covered and covered and covered ad nauseam on www.susanpowteronline.com, but for now, knowing, without a doubt, that losing lean muscle mass and water and calling it successful weight loss on any level is insane. Losing tons of weight via starvation doesn't work (that would be the 98 percent failing rate we spoke of earlier) and leaves you with a couple of horrifying side effects . . . hanging skin, feeling more exhausted than you ever thought possible, and fatter.

As I said, gastric bypass victims can tell you all about the yards of skin hanging from their bodies . . . which requires . . . ? Yes, more surgery . . . there it is, right there. Ask a gastric-bypass weight-loss patient if you can see them naked. Ask them to take their clothes off and show you the end results of that helpful little procedure. Enough said about dieting, gastric bypass, all of it . . .

Losing weight has everything to do with changing

lifestyle habits that don't work. If you do this before opting for surgery, no matter how much weight you have to lose, you won't need the surgery, and if you do it after surgery, you'll have one hell of a hard time doing what must be done to be well. When the poster girl for gastric bypass gains the weight back (and she did), she moves on to another problem.

As horrifying as rerouting internal organs to impose starvation dieting is, it's not what lured me out of my self-imposed exile. Nothing the AMA does could surprise me anymore; they don't have the power to lure me off the farm. It was, as I said, a doctor that did it, but not one of the gastric boys, no, it was a dead doctor who got me dusting off the throne and got me mad as hell. Atkins. I came back to work to stalk Atkins. Imagine my surprise when I looked up from the diaper pail and heard high-protein weight loss, not possible.

All of the above is directly connected to lifestyle. The way you are, or are not, living is connected to much more than your inability to stick with a diet, your lack of willpower, your inability to make the most basic decisions, you lazy slob. There is only one way on the planet Earth to change the way you look and feel. I said it years ago and it still applies. You have to:

eat

breathe

move and

think

You have to reclaim your body, and your brain, by doing the same things I did to lose (and never find again) over 133 pounds, the same thing thousands of people are doing right now, the same things every human body must do . . . internally change your body by externally changing your life and its style one bad lifestyle habit at a time. And before you know it, your life, your body, and your brain will reconnect because they are, directly, connected . . . another little fact that has been denied for years.

three

Oxygen

If it's your brain and body you need to reconnect, and you do, you'll need to start with step one. A step nothing is going to happen without. Oxygen. Way before "carbs vs. protein" is the most vital ingredient in wellness (and again, interestingly enough, something you never hear talked about) is oxygen. Before the food lists, before the "but what do I do about, before any of it is . . . oxygen. The only thing you can't live without for more than five minutes. If you'd like to test the theory, hold your breath for five minutes. A statement I couldn't make years ago even though it's true, all the lawyers said no can do. According to the legal experts of the past, if I said, "Hold your breath for five minutes" to make the point about oxygen being the only thing you can't live without for more than five minutes, you would. My response? Those stupid enough to, should.

Oxygen . . . without it you die, "by, Susan Powter." A big reason to get some, for sure, but not all you need to know about oxygen. Oxygen and weight loss are directly connected because:

Fat burns in oxygen.

Your metabolic rate activities in oxygen.

Oxygen feeds every cell and every muscle in the human body.

Oxygen is life.

Need more reasons? I didn't, once I made the most basic connections about oxygen, and neither will a whole lot of thinking people who may just never have thought about it and certainly hadn't heard anything about it from the health experts. You haven't heard about it because it's not being said . . . therein lies everything you need to know about how wrong everything they say is. How can you advise people about health when you leave out the most vital ingredient in wellness?

I've been talking about oxygen for too many years to think about right now, and will never, till the oxygen stops, stop talking about it. Oxygen has everything to do with burning fat, increasing strength and energy, and loving the way you look and feel. A few (and it's only a few) other simple things do, too. But let's for a moment (it only takes that long) talk about oxygen and what it can, and will, do for you.

Oxygen being as vital as it is begs the question, how to get it. There are only two ways to get oxygen into your body. Walk around with an oxygen tank and suck from it every couple of seconds, or move in it. And, exercise is connected to weight loss, wouldn't you say? This is where the "breathe" and "move" come together . . . and they do.

Movement in oxygen is how fat burns. Movement in oxygen is how your body activates in hundreds of ways. Movement in oxygen for thirty minutes or more, otherwise known as aerobic activity is the definition of aerobic. *Any* movement for thirty minutes or more in oxygen. The definition of aerobic activity . . . there's your degree, and that's about all it takes . . . shh, don't tell the physiologists.

Aerobic activity is how you are going to get oxygen into your body. Eat, you must; breathe and move, you are going to. Fat burns when you move in oxygen, so that's how you are going to burn fat. Your metabolic rate increases when you move in oxygen and your metabolic rate increases when you eat. Two things destroy metabolic rate . . . dieting and inactivity. Hasn't your doctor told you? Probably not, and why not, but the fact is . . . those are the facts. If you are suffering (as millions are) from a metabolic "issue," then at the top of the list of things you must do are eat the highest-quality foods on a regular basis and move. Activating your metabolic rate has every-thing to do with you losing weight. The way fat burns (aerobic activity) has everything to do with you losing weight. Feeding every cell and every muscle in your body what every cell and every muscle needs to live also has everything to do with you losing weight. See, it all works together. I must assume at this point in sorting out the politics of past stupid that interconnected is beginning to make much more sense.

Oxygen is the most vital ingredient in wellness, and movement in oxygen is how fat burns . . . which is how you are going to get rid of fat . . . and how that fat ended up hanging from all over your body is connected to a few more things than your willpower. The facts need to (at the very least) be considered when trying to sort out this weight "issue" of yours. Clearing up much of the confu-sion surrounding something as simple as fat is vital. You'll notice (you'll see it everywhere once you begin to see it) that the experts are always complicating very simple things. A strategy that leaves you needing an expert. Fat is as simple to understand as it gets, but you wouldn't know it with so many being so confused.

Fat

Fat is a fuel. One of the three fuels your body uses to live. That's about all you ever have to know about fat other than the fact that the human body does not manufac-ture it. Something I had to face years ago, when I weighed

260 pounds, was that there isn't a body on earth that manufactures fat. You don't go to bed one night . . . and vavoooom, 60 pounds! That's not what happened to me, and not what happened to you. That's not the way fat ends up hanging from the human body. It has to be eaten, a whole lot of it, and you have to not move for years in order for it to accumulate. If you have extra fat hanging from your back, your arms, your belly . . . wherever . . . you simply have a wholesale supply of one of the fuels your body uses. That's all. Millions of people are fat because millions of people are eating tons of fat. The average American's daily caloric fat intake is over 43 percent a day. Which means almost one half of the calories you eat a day are from fat. Way, way too many fat calories. That's what it takes to get fat, and we haven't even begun to talk about the kinds of food millions of people are eating to get that much fat in every day, which we will, because no weight-loss discussion could/should happen without talking about the toxic waste people are eating and calling food. For the moment, in the moment, let's talk fat the fuel. Fat . . . way too much of it . . . and millions of people fat . . . are you beginning to see a connection? In sticking with the gas-in-the-car theory (car can't drive without it), if you have fat hanging from all over your body, essentially you have been standing at the gas tank of life filling your tank, and you haven't gone anywhere for years. Pouring the gasoline in and not moving and?

You've got a flood. A tsunami of one of the fuels your

body uses to live. You are suffering from the simple mathematics of pouring something in and not using it up. And this particular fuel is different, not like the other two fuels your body uses . . . because fat is the fattest fuel. Have a look at another tried-and-true from back in the day, the infamous "not-all-calories-are-created-equal chart":

One gram of protein = 4 calories

One gram of carbs = 4 calories

And one gram of fat?

One gram of fat = 9 calories

One gram of fat equals nine calories, more than twice the calories of the other two fuels your body uses. More than twice. Fat is the fattest fuel.

Any connection to enormous amounts of fat consumed and no movement?

Any question there may be consequences to the lifestyle you've been living? Any confusion about what's happening to your body? Yes, there is. Interestingly enough, there is nothing *but* confusion. A bit suspect when you think about (operative word, *think*) how simple this could/should be: eat fat, get fat; don't move for years, get unwell. But it's not. Not simple to understand because you never get past the "yeah, but." Not your "yeah, but"—I mean the experts. All you hear is contradictory information, one theory vs. another, "yeah, butting" one another to death (I wish) with their sound-bited advise. The discussion never gets past the "yeah, buts," and that is not coincidence. It's the spin . . . you know what that is; watch FOX. The spin. The disconnected-from-anything-close-to-the-truth-and-nothing-but-the-whole-(not processed)-truth applies to more than food. Fractioned works in the favor of the spinners, and the sponsors of the spinners. Sponsors favor sound-bited stories "atmospherically" ingested by millions . . . after all, ingestion is ingestion.

Spend a moment in the eat crap and live like crap theory/reality. My question is no matter what the circumstances—childhood trauma, injuries, region of the country you are from—why not just try cutting back on fat if you have a ton extra hanging from your body? Why not start to move if it's been a hundred years since you have moved? And why, oh why, isn't every weight-loss discussion about eating a ton less fat and moving once in a blue moon?

Two things that could/will change everything. No need for all the other endless discussions: "My family won't touch healthy food, What about my knee injury (from 1912)?" "What do I do about protein?" "Does this require jogging, there's not time now, how oh how?" "I don't want to get bulky, where am I going to get my calcium from?"

What about? What about the lifestyle you are living right now? The politics of confusion is real. It's invisible and atmospheric; you know it. Why not change what is simple to change, starting with fat and movement, and see for yourself if those changes change anything or everything. Reread what I just said; it makes sense.

No matter what all your other issues are, two things are for sure: if you eat less fat, increasing the quality of the fuel you are putting in, and, move, you are going to change the way you look and feel. No question about it. That's absolutely true, and exactly where we are staying in this little, very interesting if I may say so myself and I may, life-changing discussion.

Go wild with me (without an expert in sight), let's agree that eating 43 % of your daily caloric intake as fat gives you a good chance of being fat. Cutting back on the amount of fat you take in, especially if you have a ton of extra hanging from your body, is a good idea. Cutting back on the amount of fat you take in and moving in oxygen to burn the extra fat you've got hanging is solution. A couple of simple human-body facts say it all, fat burns, you stop taking in a ton and start moving to burn off the ton you've got all over your body, and you get leaner.

Fat is not the problem. Fat is vitally important—essential to the human body. Fat is fuel. Fat insulates internal organs, keeps your body temperature exactly where it needs to be, and does many other things that I don't ever need to know about. What I do know and what you need to know, to understand what's been "happening" to you, is fat is not the problem. Astounding amounts of fat, gotten from the worst crap on earth, is the problem.

A couple of the problems. Glutinous amounts of one of the fuels your body uses, and no activity. Two things that are directly connected to the problems of overfat and unfit. Not a soul could disagree with that. Simple, right? Wrong. Oh, so wrong. Wrong, wrong, wrong. Say something that simple about this huge (pun-pardoning time) "issue" of obesity, and you'll get nothing but a fight from every expert on every panel in every never-ending weight-loss discussion. Say that too much fat and not enough activity are connected to overfat and unfit and all you'll hear is "yeah, but . . ."

Yeah, but what about and off they go, and they go far. All the way back to your childhood. They—the self-love, self-esteem, self-control, self-reconstruction experts—love to do this because . . . your self is the problem. That's what they want you to believe. You lazy millions of people, you. You, food addict. You no control, your willpower issue; you. You irresponsible mother, you. You, you, you.

The word *stupid* in the title of this book refers to a couple of things. One of them is how you are being treated by some mighty mega-industries and how this causes millions of not-so-stupid people to act stupid. A very, very effective technique . . . treat 'em like idiots and . . . ? Bad Parenting 101: treat them like idiots and you raise idiots. A symptom I see everywhere I look.

Every time I hear the question "Where do I start?" it confirms what I already know . . . poor things, she's been lobotomized. Millions of women have been lobotomized. Back in the day, you needed your father's and/or your husband's permission to get your lobotomy. Now it's all done biochemically, and daily. It's true, easily proven, and between you and me, no matter what the experts say, all the confusion you've felt about the question of how to get rid of fat is proof enough that something's happened to your brain.

If you want to reverse the lobotomization, here's what you need to do to burn fat fifteen extra pounds or two hundred extra pounds no difference. Start by cutting back on a fuel you obviously have way too much of: fat. Then start moving to burn the extra supply of that fuel: fat.

God forbid you should make a decision that complicated? Who do you think you are, making dietary decisions, you might die of calcium deficiency. Taking your nutrition into your own hands? Your bones will snap, you won't be well, you could make a terrible mistake, and . . . ? And what? Listen to the experts and end up in the same shape millions of others are in, that's what. I took my health, and the health of my family, into my own hands years ago, and I highly recommend that you do the same. Check with your doctor before you put one foot in front of the other . . . or do what you need to do today, before you find yourself with one foot in the grave. You are going to make a lot of healing decisions in your life for as long as you are living your life, and I mean that literally. You are going to make all nutritional decisions for your children until they are old enough to make their own . . . who the hell else is supposed to? Treat them like idiots, or expect what should be expected increasing expectations all around.

The powers that be (not for long) have been calling you stupid for years, making you feel dumb as hell (every mother in every pediatrician's office; that's all I have to say) every time you question anything, and in worked. They got you, okay, who cares? When it comes to weight loss, this is where obesity being epidemic works in my favor . . . and not in the powers that are soon not to be's favor. The very few people who are telling the truth about weight loss have an enormous opportunity when epidemic numbers of people are suffering from the same thing. Because there's got to be something more involved than millions of lazy-ass selves. It's so simple now to spotlight the contradictions, which make my life, and will make yours, much easier. You'd think with all the communicating going on (panel after panel), you would have at least gotten those two very basic life-changing facts about losing weight. Anyone who's ever done a segment on TV, one of the most pervasive mediums on earth, can tell you why you are not seeing what I'm talking about on TV. You have no idea, unless you've done one, how much of a five-minute television interview is taken up with a moronic interviewer "yeah, butting" simple facts to death. Annoying as hell for me, and horrifying for you.

Back in the day when "they" owned all the avenues of distributing information, you didn't get what you so desperately needed and I got annoyed . . . annoyed enough to never want to do it again, i.e., exile.

They can "yeah, but" saw all they want. I respond, and you get the truth. The facts are the facts and the facts will be blogged, bitched about, eaten, breathed, and moved nonstop you know where, and you will be my guests. Much more the way it should have always been, and now is. Never before could a fitness hermit (did I mention I am) come back to work, barely ever leaving the house, and still get life-changing facts to every thinking person who wants them. Beginning to see how this works?

Fact: I lost over 130 pounds, and never found them again. The only way (on earth) I'm ever going to get fat again is if:

I eat a ton of fat for a long time . . .

And . . .

I stop moving for a long time . . .

Because that's how I got fat and that's how you got fat. That's very good news if solution is what you want because it's much easier to stop eating fat and start moving than it is to solve your childhood issues and it does more good. Politics? Are you kidding? You couldn't imagine (perhaps you are beginning to see) just how pervasive the politics of keeping you completely confused about something as simple as fat is. Understanding, acknowledging what has been happening in your life for years, is as vital as "eat, breathe, move, and think." And it has everything to do with you never living stupid again . . . which, in turn, has everything to do with you loving the way you look and feel . . . which is the point. Getting past the "yeah, buts" and the "yeah, butters" is one of the biggest lifestyle X-changes you'll ever make.

Yeah, but what about:

genetics?

metabolic set-point disorders?

thyroid problems?

food addictions?

What about the relationship you have with . . . ?

What about . . . ?

What about . . . none of it? Who cares? Genetics, metabolic set-point disorders, thyroid problems, childhood horrors . . . include them if you'd like after you've spent a second accepting some simple, indisputable truths. Include them while you are taking the actions of cutting back on the fuel you have too much of, and moving. Oxygenate, activate . . . why the hell not?

The "yeah, but," without the but (I'm not even going to pardon that pun) when it comes to fat is . . . it makes you fat. Yeah, if 43 percent of your daily caloric intake is fat, it's way too much. Yeah, what people are calling food . . . isn't. You and I, staying in the "yeah" before moving on to the "but," which will dramatically decrease your butt, is where change happens. Do it, see what happens to all the other stuff. Your childhood trauma isn't going anywhere. Your fat can. See what happens to that injury when you take ninety pounds off of it. Sleep apnea . . . for God's sake, take off the boulder of weight sitting on your heart, and maybe you won't have a sleep problem, which it's not. Jesus, don't get me started. Restless legs syndrome? Way before the heavily advertised onslaught of this particular syndrome/disease, I was told by a three-hundred-plus-pound, very bright woman, on tons of meds, that she had just found out, from her doctor, she was suffering from a syndrome called restless legs syndrome. I was dumbstruck and told her so. Did I mention she was extraordinarily bright?

I suggested she try two things, two things that affect everything else . . . food and movement, two big solutions to her two big problems. Doesn't that just make sense? You'd think so, but you'd be wrong. If it made sense, wouldn't the experts in the field of health be spending all their time and energy suggesting the same things? You know why.

What they've been doing for years has worked brilliantly. It's called "iatrogenic." Create your own expertise, iatrogenic everything. Create your own need and convince millions they can't make a move without you. It's the world we live in today and it's got nothing to do with the majority . . . however, from this moment on, you will be the expert on the subject of your health. No need to call your doctor every time you make a move. No need to check with anyone but you, your intuitive common bloody sense, and activate that common sense. It will dramatically change your life.

four

Food and Movement

Let's talk about food. High fat, low quality, processed vs. real food. Let's talk about food. I have a couple of dietary rules in my home, I've had them for years.

1. If it glows in the dark, we don't eat it.

I'm not waiting for the fluorescence manufacturers to tell me their product isn't deadly because it is, done.

2. If there is one word in the ingredient list I can't pronounce, I don't buy it.

Why would I?

3. If I go into the store to buy maple syrup and I don't see the word *maple* in the ingredient list, it's not

going into my body or my (operative word, *my*) sons' bodies.

One real ingredient, there's a standard.

4. Refined white sugar, refined white flour, and refined white men are directly connected.

Especially the refined white men in the refined White House.

Four 101 food rules that affect/effect much. Huge changes can be made by you, with no expert in sight, simply by using your common sense. Now, watch as the politics and the menu plan mix, and they do. The most powerful consumer market in the massive food business is . . . ? Women. Imagine if you didn't buy:

the foods sold to you

the promises blasted at you

the flat-out lies told to you . . .

A whole lot of foods, according to my four simple rules alone, are immediately exposed. Imagine how much will change when you change what you are putting in, into your grocery cart and into your body. The ripple effect, yep, and the $276 billion food industry knows it. An educated consumer is not the goal of billion-dollar companies . . . or your health-care experts, for that matter. They are perched on very expensive, finely constructed pedestals and only one thing can knock them off. You. Here are a couple of very real lifestyle issues: food, consumer markets, massive government lobbies, huge corporations . . . never mentioned in the never-ending weight-loss discussions, and they *are* connected. Weight loss and world peace . . . oh, if only. Weight loss and war . . . there *is* a connection.

If it's war you'd like to discuss, and it seems nobody discusses anything but war, certainly these days, then let's talk about wars much closer to home. Biochemical warfare. The biochemical warfare going on in the bodies, and the brains, of millions of people. The biochemical warfare being waged (literally) by . . . ? Directed at . . . ? By our own, at our own, yep. Nothing new about blowing up our own, not at all. Beginning to see why I resent being shoved off to the side of all political discussions and late-night everything . . . oy, the eleven-thirty late-night boys' club gets tiring for the other half, meantime.

Let's agree (and move the hell on). The advertising, socializing, and glamorizing of a nearly 50 percent daily fat intake and the life "ya just gotta be living" to get over-fat and unfit is an extraordinarily well-organized, heavily funded, much-riding-on-it club. A club (guess which gender) that wields the same power as all of the other clubs have wielded for a good five thousand years. What that means to you and your daily fat intake is quite simple. You have to know, starting now, the truth. You have to know the truth and make the most basic, easy-to-do, know-it-once-and-for-all changes, starting with three things. Fat, movement, and thinking.

You have to know, from this moment on, that:

Eating a ton of fat and not moving are connected to you being overfat and unfit.

High-fat foods, for the most part, are as obvious as daylight, and you already know what most of them are.

You already have (and have had for a while) a lot of the information you need to lose weight.

You have to know that a good place to start would be to cut back, or cut out:

- tubs of soda
- deep-fried
- buttered-to-the-nines
- Creamy stuff that sits in freezer
- Doughy and gooey

Substitution lists abound.

Without knowing anything about nutrition, and you know:

A potato . . .

Cut into thin slices . . .

Is it high fat?

When those same thin slices are dumped into a vat of grease, is it high fat?

No need, at this stage of the reclaim-your-body-and-brain game, to spend any time on the enormous amounts of:

sugar

flavorings

enhancers/preservatives

Poisons, that's what the fast-food boys add to what once was a potato. And then there is the farmland they destroyed to get you such crap, and the toxic chemicals they used to manufacture it, and the cancers skyrocketing in and around (I'm talking globally) their "farmlands" and, and, and, . . . how about we just stay with high fat, and what you can do about it now and forever?

I just made potatoes. Organic baby reds, pressure-cooked for ten minutes, drained, sprinkled with sea salt, a dollop of soy sour cream (just a tad) peppered and chived, and they couldn't have been better. I did not sit down and calculate the amount of fat, protein, sugar, fiber, and everything else my potatoes had to offer. No need. What I did was eat them, over a three-bean spinach-and-tomato salad with sesame lemon dressing, and enjoyed the hell out of it.

High-fat foods are easy to spot and quite simple to cut way way back on. Eating whole, real foods is as easy as

it gets. One comes from the vats of man, usually screaming "bargain and convenient" at you. And the other?
Comes from the Mother, Nature. The foods you hear
nothing about. Not the foods being advertised at you.
Food you don't have a clue what to do with . . . and why
would you?

Grains, beans, fruits, and vegetables. By the thousands
of varieties. Bountiful. Dropping from trees, vines,
bushes. I don't pick the stuff, but I buy it. Thousands of
foods, prepared thousands of ways that you don't have to
think twice about nutritionally. The foods on the perime-
ter of your megamart. The foods you have to have to
teaching degree to get your kids to eat, according to the
corporations who make the other foods. Foods that, until
very recently, could get you arrested if you suggested they
had anything to do with anything or, God forbid, could
heal disease! Heretic, I could tell you stories, and will.

All of a sudden it turns out that whole foods have
value. Well done, Nature. Foods grown in systems that
didn't destroy the earth. Foods grown (bountifully) without dioxin. Real, whole foods. The foods you have no idea
what to do with . . . but in sticking with the most important thing (you getting the answers to your questions),
let's ask a question. One question, and you'll know everything you need to know about whether or not the food
you are eating is whole. I'll jog your memory by quoting
myself, a line from one of my infomercials years ago:
"Have you ever seen an oatmeal tree?" No, you haven't,
because oatmeal doesn't grow that way. Oatmeal isn't a
whole food. Oatmeal is, however, a very good example

that explains much about whole foods, which is the reason I'm using it. No need to go off on the should-I-or-shouldn't-I eat oatmeal "yeah, butting," go with it, you'll see, oatmeal applies to all foods.

Have you ever seen an oatmeal tree? No, you haven't because that's not how oatmeal grows. That's not a typo, that's your answer. If you ever want to know if the foods you are eating are whole, ask the question "Does it grow that way?" Hasn't it been said before, ask and ye shall? Well, ask. How does oatmeal grow? Not in flakes, and absolutely not in flakes that cook up in one minute. The original food is . . . ? A question you should ask about everything. Now, get off oatmeal.

But right now it doesn't matter. What matters is . . . pick a food, any food.

Have you ever seen a bread tree?

Have you ever seen a cereal tree?

Have you ever seen a-seven-grain-muffin tree?

Have you ever seen a Power Bar tree?

Have you ever seen a granola tree?

Have you ever seen a pasta tree?

Have you ever seen a liquid meal tree?

Increasing whole, real foods in your life has everything to do with knowing what they are. Whole foods are foods that are grown that way. As in apple on a tree, the apple.

Corn on a cob, whole. Rice, paddies are full of it. Oranges, come in groves. Beans, stalk them. Pumpkin, vined all around. Does it grow on a bush, a tree, a vine . . . from the Mother of them all, Nature? Did it grow that way? Ask the question in the privacy of your own brain, and think about it. Increasing the amounts of whole foods you eat—grains, beans, fruits, and veggies—is something you are going to do, which is going to make an astounding difference in the way you look and feel. No longer disputing, even if the experts do; what is indisputable is foundationally life changing. Agree? Good, let's move on.

Fact: You don't have to think about high fat when you are eating whole foods. You don't have to think about toxic waste when you are eating whole, real food, unless it's grown by "the highest quality" massive corporations. You don't have to think about preserved, pasteurized, and pummeled when you eat whole foods, which makes your new life a whole lot easier. Unless you are living on avocado, hearts of palm, and coconuts, you don't have to think about:

fat

fiber

water

nutrients

No need to think about any of that with thousands of varieties of whole, real foods. Because they are perfect.

"Low fat" and "grains, beans, fruits, and veggies" are synonymous. "Fiber" and "nutrient-rich," synonymous. All you have to do is get familiar with these gems of nature and eat them. The foods you need to worry about are:

enriched

preserved

flavored

enhanced

made by man

Only when the experts enrich it do you have to worry. Enhanced for you and your family, and they have enhanced disease and the girth of you and your family.

Eating more whole, real foods than processed ones pretty much guarantees that you'll reduce the hell out of your daily fat intake.

Fact: Over 65 percent of the average American's daily caloric intake is processed food.

This is where the protein boys get ya. When they say carbs, they are only talking about one kind of carb and they are not saying the word they don't want you to know. Processed foods. Whenever you hear a discussion about high-protein foods, simply substitute the word *crap* for *carbs.* Processed foods is what they are talking about and selling more of.

The other carbs? The best fuel. The lowest-fat, complex, brilliantly burning fuel, exactly. Complete carbohydrates. *Whole foods.*

Eating whole, real foods will give you (food being fuel, and it is) what you are going to need to move . . . which burns the extra, junky fuel off. Interconnected . . . because everything is. It's easy to see how sticking with human-body basics (all humans' bodies) makes things simple and quite clear, both the answers and the questions.

And my question is: What? You don't already know that? Yes, you do. You know good food from living-hell food. You know better from worse. You know you should eat vegetables. You know fruits are good. But you've been living like you don't have a clue; that's another way the high-protein boys get you. The hardest part about getting well is admitting how unwell you've allowed yourself to get, and realizing that you've known about most of the stuff that can change everything all along. Admitting you've been duped in a big way is not easy. Moments of consciousness, lightning rods to your brain . . . that, once heard, can no longer be denied . . . these are hard to face. However, face them you will by connecting one of the biggest, life-changing dots you'll ever connect. How the *stupid* happens.

The biggest detour in the history of the world.

The Eastern definition of crisis is danger and opportunity, equally. Here in the West, the Hallmark-card version is something you hear people say all the time about catastrophic situations. "I never thought I'd say this, but _____ (fill in the blank) turned out to be the best thing that ever happened to me . . ."

Growth in crisis; you've heard it.

Crisis is danger and opportunity, and overfat and unfit is a crisis. Certainly a physiological one. The opportunities in going from unwell to well are obvious . . . thousands of health benefits . . . looking and feeling much better, losing a ton of weight. The danger in you getting well is not as obvious, not spoken but, you know it. You sense it, and it's real. There isn't a much more dangerous thing a woman (especially) can do than get well. One of the most revolutionary things "any-body" can do is wellness, "by, Susan Powter." Activating your body is strewn with opportunity and danger. Because when you internally activate your body by getting lean, strong, and healthy enough to live your life in the passion and energy you were born to live in, it's a problem. Passion and energy. Put the words together . . . *passionate* . . . *energized* . . . *women!* Problem: When the world you live in is lethargic, diseased, overfat, unfit, and the people you are living in it with are acting like they are clueless . . . and you stop being those things . . . it shakes shit up.

five

The Self Lovers

The biggest detour in the history of the world is love. Love having everything to do with weight loss. After all, it's used, constantly, against you. According to the experts, love is directly connected to the reason why millions of people are so fat. Your complete lack of it.

Self-love, you don't have any.

Self-esteem . . . your esteem for yourself doesn't exist.

Emotional eater . . . love or sadness eating because of a broken love.

Love or sad eating.

Eating over a broken love.

None of it is true or none of it is the "love issue" that I am talking about. Your heart, your body, and your brain are all connected to one of the biggest disconnections you'll ever reconnect to. The reconnection of your body and brain . . . because you have been decapitated. Your brain and body have been severed by industries that profit much from your being disconnected, or at least believing you are.

"Decapitation" is literal and is one of the big reasons why you've been acting the way you've been acting. One sentence explains it all, one of those indisputable human-body truths that instantly clears the densest of fogs.

The same blood that feeds your body feeds your brain.

That's right, isn't it, Dr. Dr. The same blood that feeds your body feeds your brain. The same nutrients that feed your body feed your brain. The same lean muscle mass that activates your body activates your brain. The same internally-healthy-organed body feeds the three-pound organ (your brain) sandwiched within your skull. They are not disconnected. No, not at all. Your body and your brain are directly connected. The same oxygen-rich blood . . . or sludge feeds both. The same nutrient-rich . . . or nutrient-depleted body and brain. The same activated . . . or the same inactive body and brain. You get the point. Another one of those annoying, applies-to-everyone facts that your new activated life will be based on from now on. Simple facts that you'd never think were true if you look at the way millions of people are living, but far more understandable when you know what's happened. A total separation of the brain and body, when, in fact, they are not separate at all. Lobotomization and decapitation (welcome to your wellness universe), which begs the question:

"Why decapitate millions?" Why not? All kinds of specialists come from disconnecting a body from a brain. Oh, the specialties born from decapitating millions . . .

The "ologists" are thriving. "Treating" hundreds of diseases, never connecting the two because once they are connected, it's going to be a lot more difficult for them to fill their waiting rooms. Depression . . . it's all the rage. Everybody is. And you may be, but, if your ologist is treating you without insisting that your body be lean, strong, healthy, and well, then your ologist is an idiot. If your ologist has not thoroughly gone over every chemical, coloring, flavoring, enhancer, and enricher that you are ingesting and told you to stay the hell away from them all, then your ologist is . . .

That applies to everything. All disease, physical or mental, which are ultimately the same thing . . . because they are connected. But ologists be damned, and they will be when you stop believing what is simply unbelievable. Your getting well is the most important thing to me and not for the reasons you may think. Your body reactivating will be, in and of itself, a revolutionary change in your life, but that's not what I'm interested in. Fitness is easy. Weight loss is a given. It's embarrassingly logical, simple to do, and takes very little to maintain . . . forever. By the time you finish this book and come to live with me (did I mention that you're moving in?) at www.susanpowteronline.com, you'll be well on your way to changing everything . . . but your weight loss is not my motivation. Your body getting well is a given . . . it's your *brain* I'm interested in. Your brain activating is the reason I do what I do. Let's make the big love connection.

Love

Love is a verb. An action word. I'm not sure of any action that is more important, more loving, than you giving your body what it needs to live, daily. Self love. Yep. The action of changing your lifestyle is, in fact, one of the most loving things you'll ever do for yourself, and for those you love. You loving you is also the best way to love those you love. Love, love, love . . . see how it works.

Herein lies the danger in the biological connection to love. When your body resurrects from the living dead, your brain resurrects, the two being directly connected. When you activate your body by moving in oxygen and eating real food once in a while, your body *and* your brain activate. Your body and your brain get oxygen-rich. Your body and your brain get fed, literally, and that's very dangerous if looking around at the life you've lived, at the person you've been lying next to, at your life, at the things you've put up with . . . is frightening.

A woman named Ruth made it very clear to me one day. Sixty-plus-year-old Ruth said, "Every single thing you are saying is absolutely true, and I understand every word, but I'm not going to open those Pandora boxes in my life, Susan." My own mother died from not being willing to look at the losses . . . and from the losses. Every time I hear about the phoenix rising from the ashes, it makes me crazy. Talk about half the story. Rising from the ashes . . . stop there. Ashes . . . where did they come from? From burning. And burning hurts like hell, and it isn't fun. Burning means death, as does rising! You have to burn before you rise. That's what's never mentioned when they talk about phoenixes rising, but it's true.

When your body resurrects, so will your brain, and that's where love and decapitation come in.

Love. The old heartstrings! Your heart, filled with love. Heart, soul, love, spirit . . . ahhhh, love. Well, none of it is true. Love has nothing to do with your heart. That is flat-out not true. Your ologist knows that. Love has nothing to do with your heart. Love from your heart . . . no, you don't. "I love you so much," as you clutch your chest. Your heart has nothing to do with love. Your heart is a muscle (biochemics, biochemics), an important muscle, but a muscle all the same. Increasing cardio endurance, your heart muscle strength, is something you are going to do to burn fat, and a few other vitally important things . . . but it's got nothing to do with love. Not at all. As a matter of absolute fact, all feeling, sexuality, creativity, spirituality, all love comes from . . . ?

That three-pound organ sandwiched between your skull: your brain. Isn't that right, Dr. Dr.?

When your body gets well, your brain gets well. Danger. When you resurrect from the walking physical dead, you resurrect from the walking brain-dead. Danger. That being the absolute truth, why, oh why, do you think the experts have fractured and completely separated the sciences of healing as they have? Simple enough to answer, it's rhetorical. Always look where the profit lies. If you want the answers to a whole lot of things that affect the way you look and feel, all you ever have to do is spend a minute looking at how much money, marketing, and manpower is put toward what. Look at where all the energy is going, at the things they most don't want you to see. Clearly seeing everything they don't want you to know is simple; look at what they are trying hardest to cover up. Powerful body, powerful brain, powerful consumer market, millions of women powerful, creative, sexually, inspired, and alive . . . are you kidding? What the hell would happen to the world if millions of women were all that. Exactly, the beginning of world peace! Or the only way to world peace, "by, Susan Powter."

If you want to understand how powerful this truth is, just suggest to your health-care provider that your body and brain are connected, you'll see what happens. Regaining power—physically, mentally, and "atmospherically"—is extraordinarily healing and has nothing to do with "any-body" but you. You, reclaiming your body, your brain, and your life is one hell of a good place to start . . . starting with basic "biological facts" like love.

Self Love and Weight Loss

Love has nothing to do with burning fat. I burned over 130 pounds while I hated like poison. I didn't sort out one thing, still haven't, and I'm stronger at fifty than I was at twenty. Love has nothing to do with building lean muscle mass or increasing strength and energy. If you think I've matured an iota, you are wrong. I haven't. I hated my ex-husband twenty-five years ago and I hate him more now. He was an idiot then and he's a bigger idiot now. No "closure" . . . and I'm leaner, stronger, and healthier than I've ever been.

To be powerful physically, in your own life, and acting (*love,* an action word) power-filled in the world around you means you have to understand two things. One, how to begin the process of regaining your basic physical power, something you are well on your way to completely understanding already, and two, the definition of the word *power.*

Power

Yours. Knowing it, using it, and living (far better) in it daily is something you are going to do if you want your body and your life back. I am the only fitness expert who has the audacity to connect weight loss and world peace, and I will. You will also, once you understand what power really means, way beyond the one-dimensional box it's been presented in.

Power, according to *Webster's* means:

A position of ascendancy over others.

A one-dimensional definition and certainly what you think of when you hear the word *power.*

Another definition of the word power is:

The ability to produce an effect.

A definition worth repeating . . . the ability to produce an effect.

And when it comes to this weight issue of yours and your ability to create the effect of losing it, you've felt . . . ? Everything but powerful. Power-less. Powerless to eat better. Powerless to exercise. Why? How are millions powerless over such simple things? The truth is, it's been a while since most women I've met have felt anything close to powerful in their daily lives. How could you possibly feel powerful when you can't even "produce the effect" of something as simple as losing weight. Fail, over and over again, and it gets to you. If you can't control yourself enough to lose a bit of weight, forget about designing, implementing, and building your life. Which, when you think about it, pretty much sucks.

Another definition of the word power is:

Physical might.

Enough said. Imagine you knowing you have "the ability to produce" the effect of "physical might" in your life. And, as I've said, some of the smartest people I've ever met can't imagine it. Fascinating. Living with physical might in your life is as easy as getting oxygen into your blood, getting rid of the fat hanging from your body, and adding one absolute fact of the lose-all-the-weight-you-want-to-lose-forever matter:

Lean muscle mass.

If you want physical might in your life, you have to build it. The way you are going to do that is by building lean muscle mass, adding strength training to your daily life. And without a doubt, adding physical strength training to your life produces a whole lot of effects that change . . . everything.

six

Fat, Burning

Movement in oxygen, for thirty minutes or more, to burn fat is step one. Increasing lean muscle mass is also step one if you want to burn fat quickly, properly, and forever. Lean muscle mass is metabolically the most active tissue in the human body. Internal active tissue, you want that. Internal active tissue, lean muscle mass (not what you want to lose anymore and call successful weight loss), not a problem now that you are never dieting again. Building lean muscle mass is a must, for a whole bunch of reasons. Active tissue burns fuel. Strength begets strength. Having the muscular strength to do everything you are doing right now without the strength to do it . . . makes your life easier. Building lean muscle mass burns the hell out of fat. Lean and cut looks fabulous. Just a couple of the hundreds of reasons why you are going to build the most active tissue in the (all humans') body. Building lean muscle mass is simply a matter of picking up weight, using that weight as added resistance, and doing basic repetitions to build muscle tissue, routine after routine . . . available for you in the "Move" section of www.susanpowteronline.com. Upper body and lower body. Basic exercises . . . I've got a million of them, folks. Alternating the body parts you work, sprinkled into your aerobic routine, and you've got one hell of a workout that will change everything. Biceps, triceps, shoulders, back, chest . . . different muscle groups, three sets of ten done while you are burning the hell out of fat will ensure that you'll burn more fat.

Active tissue burns fuel, and if you've got some extra "fuel" hanging from all over your body, building active tissue will help burn that extra fat off. Problem solved. Building lean muscle mass turns a human body into an internal, fat-burning machine. But suggest building lean muscle mass to a 350-pound person or someone who is twenty pounds overweight, for that matter, and the first thing you'll hear is the "yeah, but" of lean muscle mass: "I don't want to get bulky."

Something I hear over and over again, and it's something that never ceases to amaze me, because if you are overfat, you are bulky already. Fat is wide. Fat is what's dripping over your jeans. Fat is waddy. Fat is what's hanging from your body not lean muscle mass, and if it is lean muscle mass hanging from your belly, even I suggest you run to your local emergency room and get checked out. I would never suggest anything that gives you that hideous bodybuilder look. Not for a moment would I suggest you go for the bulk most people think of when they think of building lean muscle mass. The polar opposite of anorexia is bodybuilding. Extreme dieting and exercise to attain a hideous look. What's the difference?

Building lean muscle for a leaner, stronger, healthy, fat-burning internal machine of a body has nothing to do with bulk, but fat does. Take off your clothes, turn sideways, and have a look, bulky. So don't ever worry about bulk again, because when you build lean muscle mass with me, you'll be leaner than you've ever been. If one hell of a fat-burning combo is something you want in your life—otherwise known as one of the biggest life-(very styling)-changes you'll ever make—then the combination of aerobic activity and building lean muscle mass is what you are going to do. Throw in reducing your daily fat intake and processed-food intake and . . . ? Yeah, simple and extraordinarily effective. Food and movement, I told you.

Only a detail or two to go over so you are clear, completely and forever, about what it is you are going to do to change everything.

Aerobic Activity

Fat burns in aerobic activity. As we know, the definition of the word *aerobic* is movement in oxygen for thirty minutes or more. And aerobic activity, on a regular basis, for the rest of your life is what you are going to do . . . which begs two questions. One, what does *regular* mean? And two, how do you know if you are "in" oxygen?

Human-body, aerobic fat-burning facts:

1. If you do an aerobic activity three times a week, you change nothing.

If what you saw in the mirror this morning is the way you want to look and feel, then do an aerobic activity three times a week and maintain it. If not, you might want to read on.

2. If you do an aerobic activity four times a week, you begin to change your metabolic rate.

If you are suffering from a slow metabolism, and millions are, I'm sure your doctor has told you about the two things that increase metabolism. If not, read on (fire your physician, read on, and physician, heal thyself).

3. If you do an aerobic activity five to six times a week, you burn three times the amount of fat.

If you want to lose all the weight you want to lose, these are your choices, and depending on your choices, your changes will be as much or as little as you'd like.

Maintain what you have, change your body a little bit, or burn the hell out of the fat that you don't want hanging from it. I'm going to assume you want maximum changes in your body, so I'm sticking with the six-day-a-week fat-burning prescription. After all, one half hour, six days a week, is not much to ask when you think about it.

Now, all you need to know is how to know when you're in oxygen. How to know if you are "in breath" or "out of breath" is just a matter of . . . just that. Knowing if you are in breath. "In breath" means you can breathe, finish a sentence, without huffing and puffing. If you are out of breath, you are not in oxygen. No monitoring systems necessary. No charts, graphs, pulse-taking devices strapped onto your arm (horror) . . . simply you making sure you are not:

blue in the face

sucking wind

feeling as if you are going to die . . .

If you are any of those things, you are not in oxygen. If you are any or all of those things, you are, simply, working outside of your current fitness level. Logical and simple, but . . .

I know, I know . . . panic. I absolutely know what's going through the mind of anyone who hasn't moved in a while. "How the hell do I exercise when the minute I do, I'm out of breath?" Or, "How do I get fit when I'm so unfit?" The "yeah, buts" of movement, the scrolling credits of reasons why you can't, I know.

Just another pit that you may have fallen into because not an expert in sight is talking about how the hell you are supposed to exercise. You know exercise is important, but that's about it. The basics of oxygen, fat burning, the what and how of movement, are never in the discussions . . . again, interestingly enough. As always (at least in your new lifestyle), it's quite simple. You getting fit, no matter how unfit you are now . . . in other words, wellness for everyone (said that a hundred years ago) is possible, with modification.

Increasing and decreasing your levels of intensity

At 260 pounds, I knew exercise was something I should do. I started an exercise routine a couple of times. I didn't know about oxygen, aerobic activity, cardio endurance, or modification, but I knew exercise was one of the many things on the list of must-dos. I did move . . . and I stopped because within five minutes of starting to walk, I felt like I was going to die. I went to an aerobics class at 260 pounds, in Dallas, Texas, in the eighties, in the middle of the summer, and I did almost literally die. I realized then that fitness was only for the very very fit.

At 260 pounds, I was out of breath because I had:

an enormous amount of fat hanging from all over my body

no lean muscle mass

no cardio endurance

I was unfit. Which meant? Modify. Move within your fitness level. You can move no matter what your fitness level, by moving *within* your fitness level, even if it barely exists. (Another necessary reread.)

No matter what your fitness level is or isn't, you are going to move within it by understanding a very important concept: *slow the hell down.* That's right, slow down. Or, speed up. Decreasing or increasing your levels of intensity . . . and you'll have to do this. Every day, for the rest of your well life, you are going to have to work within different energy levels for a trillion reasons. "What you ate the night before," "about to get your period," "had a fight with," or "haven't moved in forever," it makes no difference. You can increase or decrease your levels of intensity by slowing down or speeding up.

I was walking around the block in Garland, Texas, back in the day, and I started sucking wind five minutes in. I slowed down and kept walking for thirty minutes. The next day I did the same thing. Went for a walk, and when I started huffing and puffing, I slowed down and kept walking . . . and guess what happened? Within days, I noticed it took longer and longer to be out of breath. It's called building a cardio endurance level, and you have to do it. Then fat started to burn, because it does, and it was a whole lot easier moving without a ton of extra fat hanging off me, and once I started to use muscles that I hadn't used in years, they got stronger . . . which made it easier to move.

Very soon movement will be easy for you, but the most important thing for now is to move *in oxygen,* and you have to know how. The minute you are out of breath, you are going to slow down and keep walking. The minute you are out of breath, you are going to come out of the pose (yoga with me; you'll be doing it), shake it out, get your breath back, and go back into the pose. The minute you are out of breath, modification applies to everything. Staying in oxygen for thirty minutes, forty-five minutes (why the hell not add fifteen to your routine? there's a bumper sticker!), means you will get all the benefits of movement in oxygen (and you can't imagine them till you do it) and, most important, you'll be able to and want to do it again.

Not having the aerobic crap slapped out of you works best if it's something you want to be inspired to do again. You are going to be burning fat and building strength, two fabulous, new, life-changing additions to your life, and imagine if you also go wild and take in less high-fat processed crap and poison and add (here's the wild part) more real, whole foods! Solution to more than you could ever imagine possible.

Weight-Loss Prescription

What? Aerobic activity. How much? Thirty minutes a day. How often? Six days a week.

What? Build lean muscle mass. How often? Fifteen minutes a day, six days a week, at the end of your thirty-minute aerobic activity. Which gives you one hell of a workout routine. Forty-five minutes, aerobics and strength building, six days a week, for the rest of your life is the truth about fat burning, the work of working it off, and the only way it happens. If you have fat to burn, you want the best results. If you'd like to change the way you look and feel forever, you'd want to burn three times the amount of fat, wouldn't you? There is nothing more encouraging than getting results from your work. If you are unwell, you'll want to do the most you can for a lot of reasons. What you don't want to do is the very least. If you are unwell, you are in dangerous health . . . why aren't health professionals prescribing maximum lifestyle changes? From now on, assume that every question I ask about health professionals is rhetorical.

Simple and logical does not simple and logical make, not when it comes to you exercising. All I have to say to most people is you have to exercise five to six days a week for forty-five minutes (just added fifteen minutes of oxygen getting) . . . and they are out. Can't do it. Impossible. Not going to happen. You doing something five to six times a week for thirty minutes for . . . the rest of your life? Yeah-but, yeah-but, yeah-but, yeah-but . . . I know.

Interesting, a suggestion of four and a half hours a week to change your life activates total panic because there's two things you need before you could possibly dedicate four hours a week to *you*. Motivation and time. Right? You've been looking everywhere for both and you've been promised both are "out there somewhere." A bad Disney theme song, redundant, and exactly what you've been doing.

seven

Motivation and Time Management

The number one question I get, hands down, is "Where did you find the motivation to lose over 130 pounds?" The next question is "How do you stay motivated?" How did you get, where did you find, where oh where is the motivation? Three questions, but really just one. And the answer is, I didn't. I didn't find the motivation to lose over 130 pounds, and you will never find motivation. You haven't found it yet, and it's not as if you haven't been looking. Finding the motivation to _____ (fill in the blank) is never going to happen because it's not waiting anywhere to be found. You've been looking for motivation for how many years?

Looking to find the one thing you need in order to do

everything you know you should do. You just need to be motivated by some motivation that you are going to find somewhere one day? You've found it a couple of times . . . it's not as if you've never been motivated. Every time you are done with this fat thing—usually the Monday after a weekend binge—and . . . ? Every time you believed (because you were sold) that you had found the system, the plan, the combination of, you've been motivated. Then you fail right, because you lose the motivation to stick with it? You had it for a minute, and it's gone. Motivation evaporation every time.

You, you, you can't find it or keep it. Must be something wrong with your:

willpower

discipline

self-control

self-esteem

Self-flogging is what it is, and self-flogging is where they want you. You may have thought that went out with Hildegard, but it's not true, it's still all the rage. You can't stay motivated to save your life. You, you, you (again) . . . what's the matter with *you*? Dieting . . . with it's 98 percent failure rate (*all* diets) . . . and still they have you blaming yourself. Brilliantly done, wouldn't you say?

Well, the fact is, when it comes to motivation (and everything else), there is no way you are the only problem, and the politics of that stupid is becoming crystal clear by the moment. If you were the only problem, you'd be the only unmotivated person alive or a part of a very small group of motivationally incapable people, but you aren't. It seems that there are millions of people who can't find, don't have, aren't able to hang on to for the life of them, motivation. And it's not as if motivational advice, theories, beliefs, practices, and experts aren't plentiful.

Motivational speaker, I am. Known to motivate, I am. And I begin every motivational speech saying it doesn't exist. Motivation exists, but not anywhere you've been told (sold) it is. There is only one place motivation is, and it's bountiful. As much motivation as you will want or need is waiting for you. Not to bump into it . . . to tap into it. All the motivation you'll ever need is found in the process of *doing* . . . because motivation *is* in the process of doing. Something that is worth repeating fifty times. Motivation is in the process of doing, period, the end. Whatever it is, doing it is where the motivation is.

If it's wellness motivation you've been looking for, then do well things and you'll be very motivated to do more well things. Doing well things for your body and brain is where all the motivation to keep doing well things is. If it's motivated to lose weight you are dying to be, then do things that make you lose weight. Eat well. Move. Build lean muscle mass—all fat-burning things. If it's inspired you want to be in your life, do inspiring things. Motivation begets motivation. Spend a moment on the *physiology* of motivation, please. Why not? You get nothing but *psychology*, which is exactly how they keep you there.

The physical fact of the motivation matter is an unwell body (all unwell bodies) is . . .

An unwell body is a body that isn't going to be motivated to get up and move. Mine wasn't at 260. I was motivated *not* to move. A ton of fat, no lean muscle mass to speak of, and the cardio endurance of a gerbil? Why would my unwell body wake up and want to go jogging? It wouldn't and it didn't. It makes perfect sense, and again, the endless discussions discussing nothing, you only ever hearing how lazy, unmotivated, weak, out of control (I love that one) you must be to "let yourself go like you have," little lady. When, in fact, your lack of motivation is connected to quite a few very real things. Never included in the discussions because why would they want to include the whole story?

A body that is oxygen deprived will not be motivated to move. A body that is nutritionally deprived is not motivated to move. A body that has very little lean muscle mass and the metabolic activation of a slug is motivated to be sluggy. Why all the psychology and never the physiology? Something you should take up with your psychologist because the two are connected, Dr. Dr.

The way you are going to get all the motivation you'll ever need is, stop waiting for it. You are no longer going to wait until you are motivated to move, to move. When you first start this wellness thing, you will not be motivated to exercise, but you are going to move in oxygen for thirty minutes anyway. You may not be inspired to lift weights and build lean muscle mass, but you are going to build lean muscle mass anyway. I'd be glad to bet that you'll be inspired to do it with me, so begin with me whether you are motivated or not. Then you are going to do it again, and again and again, and very soon you'll be motivated in more ways than you ever thought possible.

Wellness Success

The moment you eat, breathe, move, and think with me, you will get immediate results, because fitness is immediate. The results of fitness are immediate if you know what you are looking for, and have nothing to do with what you've been brainwashed into believing are successful results.

The results of moving in oxygen are immediate. As soon as you begin to do it, you have a bit more energy. Oxygen equals energy, oxygen equals life, and when you oxygenate your blood and that blood carries oxygen to every cell and muscle in your body, you feel better. The sigh, the "Oy, I feel better" . . . it happens every time. Only one of the thousands of successful results from thirty minutes of movement. Very good return on a very small investment. Atmospheric global bank, oh I will, because it is.

Eating works the same way when you think about it . . .

Dieting is not fun. Dieting doesn't work. Dieting makes you weak, fatter, sick, not motivated to do anything, and when you try to add torturous exercise to starvation all the while you're struggling to find the time and motivation to do it all is impossible. No wonder you aren't motivated to do it . . . it sucks. Common bloody sense . . . the physiology, please. Move in oxygen today and you'll have more energy/oxygen than you had yesterday, which is an immediate result when you think about it. And that's exactly what you are going to do . . . think about it. The results of building lean muscle mass are immediate, a bit more strength and energy every time you do it. Not to mention, twist my arm, that you burn the hell out of fat when you do it. The results of eating real foods are also immediate; you feel less like shit when you don't eat shit. Day after day of doing well things, you are going to think about:

what you did

how you feel

if you think it would make your life better if you did it again

I'm talking about thirty minutes a day or an hour tops. Oh, watch me, you'll be begging for a one-hour exercise routine by the end of this book, but the point is you are going to crack that nut of motivation, and you'll have all the motivation you ever needed by asking yourself three questions every time you do eat, breathe, move, and think. It's the new (and much improved, because it works) measure of success, the only measure of success from now on. Every time you X-change a high-fat, processed, inactive, nonthinking lifestyle habit for a far more styling (life-styling) life habit, you are going to ask yourself three questions:

1. Do I feel better?

After thirty minutes in oxygen, the answer will always be yes. Thousands and thousands of classes later, never once have I heard, "Damn it, I wish I hadn't done that," or, "That was a complete waste of my damn time." You'll never get up from a meal of whole, real, nutrient-rich food and say you don't feel better than you did when you ate junk.

The next question you are going to ask yourself every time do well things for yourself is:

2. Do I have more energy? The answer will, always, be yes.

You sure as hell will have more energy if you:

get oxygen into your body

build an ounce of lean muscle mass

and eat real foods . . .

Who would be stupid enough to argue with that?
And the third question you can ask yourself is:

3. Am I shrinking?

If you eat, breathe, move, and think, you will shrink. Oh my God, what a brilliant bumper sticker! Is someone collecting these? Shrinking is the best indicator that you are burning fat, which is exactly what you want to do. No need to even say the word *scale* yet. From now on, if you want to know what successful weight loss is, a tape measure will tell you everything you need to know. Fat burns, you shrink because fat is wide, fat is waddy, and lean is lean.

Shrinking is success measured in inches gone. The clothing-size rack has more to do with the measurement of successful weight loss than any scale ever has. Clothing sizes dropping and oh, what fun that is! Burned off. The scale, okay, I'll mention it. "Scale stupid" is something I talked about years ago, but let me refresh your memory: Looking at a number on the scale to measure weight-loss success is as dumb as checking the oil of your car by looking at the upholstery. One doesn't have anything to do with the other. Especially the numbers touted as success on some of the most popular weight-loss shows . . . it makes me crazy; it is stunningly hard to be me sometimes, really.

Just like everything else, every chart, every graph, every body-type expert opinion, the scale is wrong. Lean, strong, healthy, and well cannot be measured (and isn't) on a scale. Internally activating your body, the only way to lose all the weight you want to lose and never find again, cannot be measured on that horrifying piece of bondage equipment, and that's an insult to bondage.

Your scale measures lean muscle mass, not numbers

dropped, and lean muscle mass is essential for weight loss. The scale has no number for energy, and wellness gives you more energy than you may ever have imagined possible. The scale certainly can't measure passion. If it did, it would be illegal. Passion, energy, strength . . . don't have numbers on a scale, and that's the point. All the scales do is measure what the scale makers want you to focus on . . . and it's not success.

Your doctor knows that and you might want to remind him/her of it the next time he/she tries to weigh you. There are only two things you need to do with your scale: one, give it to someone you hate, and two, never get on it again.

All the motivation you'll ever need, organically recycled (it begets itself), is available when you start doing well things on a regular basis for the rest of your life. Easy to understand . . . and yet it's still almost impossible for you to understand just how the hell you are going to do it. How you are going to do anything, especially exercise, on a regular basis for the rest of your life is confusing to millions? Even if the motivation is possible, there's another "issue" millions of people to face . . . Interesting, isn't it? The same issue . . . for *millions*?

That issue is time.

Time Management

Time, like motivation, is something you've been looking for everywhere . . . more of it. Much, much more, because if you could find (same language) the time you would certainly start doing a whole lot of things you know you should be doing . . . if only you could find the time. Time and looking for more of it is another one of those very well-planned detours. A detour that has millions of people looking for something that doesn't exist. More time in your own life, for your life.

Listen to the language, ladies. Time management. Unabashed in the language that describes what you are looking for. Time management . . . as if there is such a thing! My peers in the motivational-speaker world would have you believing that time can be managed. I'm here to tell you it can't. Time management is a misnomer. You cannot manage time. We all have the same twenty-four hours in a day, and you'd think with your life being made so convenient for you, you would have nothing but extra time. Not true. Not true at all. What is true is, most women are buried alive in their lives, looking everywhere for more time and killing themselves waiting to find it. Your finding the time *in* your life, *for* your life, is not happening and never will . . . because you can't manage time. You can't manage time, but you can manage you.

Managing your life, your needs, your body, within the same twenty-four hours we all have, is a solution for much and absolutely connected to how you do, or don't, look and feel. I had to admit back in my overfat and unfit day that there were: people who had children, and exercised, lean, strong women who had idiots for ex-husbands. There were one or two people living in Garland who ate well, and guess what, they looked good. A whole lot better than I was looking and feeling. There was one major difference between me and them and it wasn't that they had more than twenty-four hours in the day. The difference was that they were doing a few things, no matter what the circumstances of their life, that I wasn't. It dawned (lightning-bolt moment) on me that life wasn't going anywhere . . . until it went. And many days, most days, sometimes years of days, were hell. Living is hard, but it's still the best bet. Enough said; living was for me. I realized in that moment that doing a few things for myself, while life goes on, those things make life:

easier

leaner (synonymous)

stronger (synonymous)

better

I've been fit and I have been fat . . . and fit is better. Waking up every day with a foundation of wellness makes life a lot easier, and you, waiting to find the time to do the very few simple things that you must do in order to make your life a whole lot easier is nuts. You can't manage time. It is a management matter, but not anything close to what the experts in the field of time management insist it is.

The fact of the as-much-time-as-you-need-to-change-the-way-you-look-and-feel-forever matter is: How you manage you daily, your life, definitely the eat, breathe, move, and think of your life, is how you are going to have plenty of extra time. Motivation happens in the process of doing, and more time is the result. You managing your life? Your life's priorities. You doing the managing of your life, yourself within the same twenty-four hours we all have is how you:

change your body

change your health

get all the time you need to lose as much weight as you want to lose

Starting with a few basic changes in your use of time, the first being to stop asking for more time. First, there isn't any more time—take that from me, fifty years old, three kids and a life later, I can promise you I haven't found more time. Second, who are you asking? Finding the time to _____ (fill in the blank) Krazy Glues millions into not doing a thing. It's one of the big reasons why you just can't get a grip on this weight thing. "When I find the time, I will." "As soon as I have the time, I'm going to . . ." I said it, you say it, millions are saying it right now. At 260 pounds, I said it. After I work the three jobs I'm working, take care of my elderly parents, be a friend, lover, wife, and mother to the world, I'll carve out some time for me . . . after I find it, that is. And . . . it never happens.

It never happens for a couple of reasons. You've been sent (again) looking for something that is not there, and trying to find more time to tack life-changing lifestyle habits onto everything you are already doing is impossible. Overwhelmed is overwhelmed, and millions are. And the reason you are is that you are on the wrong end of an endless list. Step one in time management: Something's gotta go and it's about to . . . actually, a whole lot of somethings. Time management, the misnomer in a discussion that goes way beyond tacking *yourself* onto the endless list of all the things you have to do . . . no, no, that was my mother—not me and not you. Dead at fifty-two, did I mention?

You'll have plenty of time to work on your body because you are about to do a whole lot more than carve a minute or two for yourself . . . you are about to carve a good chunk of time out for yourself *every* day. You are going to take one hour a day. Yep, one whole, to-yourself hour a day. Figure it out, it's only an hour . . . you've got another twenty-three to do whatever you want with. One hour a day, six days a week. Grab the smelling salts for millions of women—I know what a reaction that statement creates. Six hours a week for you, in *your* life—impossible! All you need to do is reread what I just said in order to understand everything I'm talking about. Gasp at the suggestion of spending six hours a week all you want, but this is what you get:

looking and feeling better than you have in years

giving your body what it needs to live

solving the problems of overfat and unfit forever . . .

And a whole lot more . . . point being . . .
Six hours . . . I want you for one hour a day, six days a

week, for three months. If at the end of that three months, you don't like what you see, go back to your old ways. Not too much to ask; after all, it's *your* life. Added to the list? Not anymore. You are about to do something much worse than that . . . you are about to sin. And you are about to sin big, and mortally if you are a woman. You are about to put *you* first, for three months, no need to get the flogging gear out, not yet anyway.

For the next three months of your life, before anyone or anything, comes you. If you want to reclaim your body, your health, and a whole lot more, that's exactly what you have to do. Make your body, your health, and your life the top priority. Work the project, like you work all the other projects. Take care of yourself like you take care of . . . how many people? If someone you love is unwell, what do you do? Yeah. That's the point, and I don't even have to type it, you know it . . . Put the same energy into you, you first . . . horror, you selfish woman, you!

Now, about that time you can't seem to find. Step one: Stop looking for it. Step two: X-change selfless for selfish.

Full of self. Why the hell not, literally . . . and not rhetorically . . . I mean why the hell not? Full of self while you heal and restore your self back to yourself . . . it makes perfect sense. Your life, your needs, your health, your body, your brain, *you*. First. Three months, you and me at www.susanpowteronline.com. No more looking for, asking, squeezing in time for you. Demand the time in your life, for your life, and you'll find a lot more than time.

Fact: You've got twenty-four hours in a day. What you do within those twenty-four hours is going to give you the energy and strength you need to do all the other things you are doing in those twenty-four hours. Full of self is as far from unloving as you could possibly get, even though it's been presented ass-backward. The most loving thing you can do for you is you, and the most loving thing you can do for everyone is you. Love being interconnected—everything is—and love being an action, and it is. What's gotta go is you throwing away your time on everything and everybody else but you first. The truth is, it's you who's been wasting very precious time if you are overfat and unfit.

Fitness is dangerous; that's been established. You managing you is extremely dangerous because you start to love it, and you start to consider your time (especially time away from you) precious. What a thought . . . millions of women taking their energy and time seriously; God knows what will happen when that does. What happened to me, what has happened to every woman I've ever taught in every class—and that's one hell of a market-research statistic—is, I started to love that hour for me. You have no idea how dangerous (and how much opportunity) six hours a week to yourself can be until you do it.

Very soon into oxygenating your body, you will start to love the way you feel when your body is oxygen-rich. The minute your body builds an ounce of strength, you are going to love feeling stronger. Burning fat, shrinking, is one of the most exciting things on earth. Call me "surfacey," go right ahead, I still clearly remember the landmark shrinking stages as I burned the fat off my body . . . and it's been years. I said it in the first infomercial: One of the best days of my life happened at a mall. Double stroller (that was back in the day when nobody was having babies, now?), double diaper bag, exhausted, strolling the kids around because I had nothing else to do, and I was losing my mind (and oh, what a thrill a mall is for me) when it dawned on me that for the first time in forever, my thighs were not rubbing together. Remember when I ducked my head and looked between my legs on national TV . . . because I did. To this day, I remember when my belly went from three rolls to one! Oh my God, stunning. Oh, I absolutely remember when there wasn't even enough fat to grab, just the last bit of fat to burn before a tight, flat stomach. Thrilling, and I loved it. I still do. As will you. You will love getting well, and very soon into your program, you won't like it when your time is taken away from you. Not at all. After all, I'm only talking about six hours a week, and it's easily found when you take a gander at how much time you waste:

> talking to people you can't stand 'cause you can't say no

> helping the world because you think you should

> supporting _____ (fill in that blank).

All of it is fine if that's what you want to do, somebody's got to . . . but not until you are well. Fair enough. When you are strong enough to carry the weight of the bloody world, go right ahead. When you've dumped the extra weight hanging from your body, you can pick up as much "atmospheric" weight as you'd like, but until then it's killing you. I mean this literally. Knock yourself out in being kind to others when you are healthy and well . . . you'll be far more effective then anyway, and you'll love the way you look and feel while you are doing it, social work by, "Susan Powter."

The politics of selfish women . . . oh my God. A whole lot changes when women stop running around accommodating everything and everybody, and one of the biggest changes is that you'll find some of the time you've been looking for and you will never give it up again.

Your new life can begin the minute you know your energy, strength, and time will no longer be spent looking for things that are not out there (because, they aren't). Then you take the actions (*love* is an action word) and do the things that give you back . . . your body, your brain, and your life . . . and you'll have more energy and strength to live your life. Certainly, a better use of time than looking for it.

Easy to understand, but still the question is . . . how? Sure, you are going to be ready to do whatever, you'll be motivated as hell while you are reading this—why wouldn't you be?—but what's going to happen next Thursday when you are late again for everything, pissed off, exhausted, trying to figure it all out within the avalanche of your life, and one hour is as impossible as it's been for . . . how many years? How are you going to do it? If ever there was a lifestyle X-change program, it's here and now in four little words, here's how you are going to find everything including the time in your life for the time of your life.

Consciousness, honesty, behavior, and *responsibility.* Not just words (ever with me) anymore. Four words that are about to be lifejackets in your daily living. It's true . . . knowledge that is about to become (and it's quite becoming) the most powerful moments of your new lean, strong, healthy new life.

eight

Consciousness

Consciousness is an integral part of your program. As a matter of fact, it *is* the program. Consciousness, honesty, behavior, and responsibility.

Stop the Insanity explained the foundations of wellness; they never change and I'll never stop talking about them. Consider eat, breathe, move, and think the tools you are going to use to change the way you look and feel. Consciousness, honesty, behavior, and responsibility . . . your program. Certainly this program is about how you are going to do it—how you are going to change what you eat, how you are going to change whether or not you ever move, how you are going to change a lifestyle that isn't working for one that absolutely does. It's what you've been missing. Again (and again) it's not as if you don't know what total crap is. You certainly know that exercise is something that should be done, but . . . ? Exactly. Consciously, honestly, behaviorally, and responsibly is how you are going to change everything, and absolutely how you are going to change the way you look and feel.

The Politics of Stupid is all about you knowing why. Four words that are about to become tangible, applicable, and attainable in your life, four words that multiply, because consciousness begets consciousness— danger, Will Robinson. Doing "well things" begets doing well things—danger, Will Robinson. Fear and weight loss . . . they are connected. Fear—one of the big reasons why millions of women are not reclaiming their bodies, their brains . . . which is ultimately their health. Real fear, not the old (and tired) psychology of "hiding behind the fat, blah, blah, blah." I'm talking about real fear, the truth behind why a woman changing her lifestyle, completely and absolutely, is frightening as hell.

Consciousness is the first word in your lifestyle X-change program. My body didn't manufacture the extra 130 pounds that was hanging from it; this was something I had to face years ago, and the way I faced it was by getting conscious. Because, it turns out, I was completely unconscious. Running a home, raising two babies alone, working two jobs (redundant). It makes me want to go back into exile. I was unconscious. As unconscious as you are . . . and you are. If you are overfat and unfit, you are unconscious. You may be thinking what I thought when I first heard, "Screw you: I may be a little on the heavy side and not exactly loving the way I look and feel, but unconscious . . . ?" Yes, unconscious—even though you may be Ms. Millennium.

Living Your Life

Making your own money and decisions, dating, marrying, divorcing (my pattern) whomever you choose. You might even be naturopathic or holistic. There's no question that you're on the go, cell phone embedded in your ear, hybrid car double-parked as you run around like a lunatic. Still, the fact of the overfat and unfit matter is:

At 260 pounds, I was a woman living her life unconsciously. I was 260 pounds and taking care of everyone and everything. The wife was really busy constantly . . . talk about an energy suck. The friends were being befriended, the children were being loved, the home was homey . . . and my body, my life? Your body, your life? The truth is, if you were conscious, you wouldn't be doing half the things you are doing consciously . . . like feeding your body poison? Not possible. "Consciously" feeding your kids foods that cause cancer? Absolutely not. "Conscious" and destroying your earth? Yes. That's exactly what's happening.

The definition of the word (always) explains it quite clearly.

Conscious: Awake.

I was awake doing everything that needed to be done, but conscious I wasn't, because, as usual, there's more to the story. Another definition of the word *conscious* is what stopped me in my 260-pound tracks, and that definition is: intentional.

Intentional? Not 260 pounds. Ask and you shall receive. Intentional . . . the way you look and feel right now is intentional? Your intention was forty, seventy, one hundred pounds overweight by the age of . . . ? No, it wasn't intentional, because that's not anybody's intention. My intention never was "to be as close to three hundred pounds as I could get." Unwell is not intentional. Nobody designs overfat and unfit. And if your body (which dramatically affects your daily life) is not your intention, you might want to ask the question "Who's doing the intending in your life?"

Overfat and unfit is not anyone's intention. Nobody writes on the list of what they want in life: "exhausted, overfat, halfway on my way to heart disease by the time I'm thirty." No. The most conscious people I know are zombies when it comes to their health, amazingly true for millions. Why? And about the foods your kids are eating, the stuff that glows in the dark? You *intentionally* feed them fluorescent? You believe that's good for them? That's what you intentionally pick to feed the people you love most in the world? It's easy to go way beyond fitness with this conscious thing, and I will. Your relationship? When you were dreaming of your "soul mate," of the love, intimacy, and support of your dreams? Is that what you woke up next to this morning? And air you breathe? Your intention was polluted? Is this the world you intended?

Wellness getting global by the second . . . because consciousness (and wellness) is. I've never met a woman who intends destruction.

Your body, the health you are not in, and the condition of the planet are far more connected than you may have ever thought, and certainly more connected than anyone is talking about.

If you believed you could be lean, strong, healthy, and well, that's what you'd choose. The fact is, you no longer believe you can, not anymore. "It" worked. Somewhere along the line of your life (style), you stopped believing you could do anything about the way you look and feel. You've learned to live with, excuse, and justify your body. The billions of dollars spent affected you. You've accepted the powerlessness of never being able to figure this complicated weight-loss thing out, and you are stuck. Living in the symptoms, running around and around on the wheel of a lifestyle invented by . . . ? Solving the problems of overfat and unfit seem much more difficult than the instant promises and quick fixes (that fix nothing) thrown at you from every direction, but believe me, it isn't. There is nothing easy about the way millions are living. Fat isn't easy. Exhausted isn't easy. Sick isn't easy. Feeling out of control isn't easy. Failing over and over again isn't easy, and all of it does a whole lot of damage. As far as I'm concerned, this is where your program really begins . . . with four words that are about to free you. Four words that explain the Politics of Stupid better than anything: *Consciousness, Honesty, Behavior,* and *Responsibility.*

Knowledge is power?

Another lie from my motivational-speaker peers; you've heard it over and over again . . . knowledge is power. All the information in the world cannot change a thing if you don't know how to make it tangible in your daily life. America is the most statistics- and document-laden country in the world, all the charts and graphs you'd ever want to know from are available to you. They always have been and . . . ? It hasn't changed a thing . . . which means knowledge is not power. Only one of the things I love about my work is how simple it is to clear it all up when you think about it.

If your intention is not overfat, unfit, exhausted, and hating the way you look and feel, yet you are still all those things; then your body (and your brain; they are connected) is in an unconscious state, and it is. Would it be presumptuous of me to say your intention is energy, and looking and feeling fabulous? Right? If that's your intention and you are not living your life intentionally, then it's time to get intentional in, and about, your life. There is a way (this program) to wake from the unwell coma; simply get conscious.

Intentional

Intentional is you making your intentions loud and clear to you and result, you are going to do just that in three easy steps. Constantly, especially in the beginning of resurrecting from the living dead, you are going to:

remember

remind, and

redo

Another corny but true fitness moment. Don't tell the infomercial boys, but the truth is that your life can change in one minute. Change a choice, change a life, "by, Susan Powter." As true as it is, it's not something I'd hand to any late-night-sell boy. Can you imagine what they'd do with that! Which doesn't change the fact that it is the truth.

Your whole life will change . . . as a matter of fact, it's the only way to change anything . . . in one minute. X-ing out a lifestyle that isn't working for a style of life that absolutely does. And it all happens in a whole bunch of one-minute increments. One high-fat, processed, junk-food choice at a time. One inactive-to-active minute at a time. One weak-to-strong, half-dead-to-alive X-change at a time. X-ing out what isn't working for what does . . . your program! It's the only way, so you may as well start doing it today . . . talk about a bumper sticker! You are going to eat, breathe, move, and think your way back to a life of energy and strength by doing three things every time you do those four things. One minute, and for a minute, sixty whole seconds, you are going to stop and:

remember

remind, and

redo

remember

you just did, active

remember

you used to do, inactive

remember

you just burned fat

remember it's fat you want to burn

remember

you just built strength

remember

it's strength you want to build . . .

Certainly a much more productive thing to do than looking for the motivation, time, and energy you used to walk around looking for. A far better use of time, exactly . . .

Three things: remember, remind, and redo. After you've moved in oxygen for thirty minutes, spend a minute, for a minute, reminding yourself:

Inactive to active is a huge lifestyle change, but not if you don't remember. All interconnected, because everything is. One minute, and for a minute after you exercise, you are going to:

Remind

Remind yourself what it is you really want. Lean, strong, healthy, and well. Remind yourself what your intentions are, little lady. Logical; nothing complicated about it and not much to ask of yourself. One minute "to root in" new and much improved very styling life habits. And without an expert in sight, major lifestyle changes happening in the privacy of your own brain—danger, Will Robinson, danger. And it is. You running your intentional list in an activated body is filled with land mines. A method to the madness? Yep, you bet. Blood pumping, oxygen-rich, body- and brain-activated, what better time to root in . . . everything. The physiology of it all is very powerful, only one of the reasons for all the detours. You, programming new ticker-tape material into your activated body and brain, eating, breathing, moving, and thinking, all the while remembering, reminding, and redoing . . . what's not going to work about that?

I'm sticking with exercise, but it's not difficult to see how remember, remind, and redo applies to everything.

Within, what has turned into a very powerful moment in time, one minute after you do well things, you are going to remember, remind, and . . .

Redo

Inactive for active . . .

Remembering and reminding yourself. That is what you are going to do for the rest of your life. Redoing more than just your body. It could, and will, go on forever . . . the script is yours to write; that's the point. You've got four categories—eat, breathe, move, and think—to take quite a few one-minute moments every time you do what every human body has to do to get well. X-changing what doesn't work for what does.

When you get up from a meal of whole, real food . . .

Remember

You just ate real . . .

You just gave your body nutrient-rich fuel.

Remind

Remind yourself how you used to feel when you ate horrifying food. Remind yourself of the end results of disgusting food . . . look in the mirror. When you X out crap food for real food, you've done more than any diet ever could. Redoing poison for real food has everything to do with weight loss and some. Redoing the old lifestyle habit of you working against what you want in your life for the new, very stylish reality of looking and feeling fabulous. Remembering, reminding, and redoing.

It's easy to see how this works, and it does. It's real lifestyle-changing therapy, biochemical therapy. Why not? Everyone else has a bloody therapy. Remembering, reminding, and redoing your body is one of the most therapeutic things you'll ever do. Consider your lifestyle X-change program your new therapy from this moment forward . . . ISM Therapy . . . Susanism.

Remember, remind, and redo applies. One minute after moving in oxygen for thirty minutes or more, remind yourself what it felt like every time you said you were going to exercise and didn't. Remind yourself what failure felt like and remember what you feel like, at this moment, having just succeeded.

Redoing your thinking for the next time you are going to move, tomorrow. Redoing all the reasons why you just haven't been able to, redoing excuses for truth. Exercise is simple to do, it doesn't take a lot of time, and is one of the best returns on any investment you'll ever make. Remember that. Remember how you feel after thirty minutes in oxygen! Remind yourself that you are getting far better returns than what you've spent a ton of money, time, energy, and faith on in the past.

Tell the truth, and there's nothing easy about it. The hardest part of getting well is admitting how unwell you really are, it'll take the breath out of you, and then you put more than the breath back in, and, done. From this moment on, your life begins one life-changing X-change at a time, because the past does not equal the future (unless you don't change the present), never more true than when you are coming out of the overfat and unfit coma. If your intentions from this moment on are:

lean

strong

healthy, and

well . . . then here's what you are going to do.

As you are doing well things, eating, breathing, moving, and thinking your way back to a life of energy and strength, you are going to do it consciously by remembering, reminding, and redoing basic lifestyle habits, and the way you are going to do that is by making your life your intention. You, getting conscious (intentional) about something as vital as the quality of your daily life. And there's no chance of that happening without you getting honest first . . . because you haven't been.

nine

Honesty

Honesty is the second word in your lifestyle X-change program because honestly, you haven't been. You may be the most upstanding citizen on the planet Earth, but if you are overfat, unfit, and not well, you have not been being honest, and it's not as if you haven't been given every out under the sun.

Let me guess some of the reasons why you are overfat.

thyroid

metabolism

children

stress

genetics

C-section

addicted to food

thick blood

"My whole family is pear-shaped, so there's nothing I can do . . ."

The whole family may be pear-shaped, but you don't have to be the fattest pear in the orchard, or wherever pears grow, and about your malfunctioning thyroid . . . ? Honestly, when is the last time you did anything to promote glandular health?

Genetics. Yes genetics play a part in everything, but not so much in the way you look and feel as, yep, lifestyle.

Fact: Don't ever forget that 85 percent of all diseases can be directly attributed to lifestyle. Another one of those annoying little facts, straight from the AMA, but is it ever heard? It's not, because when you think about it, 85 percent is a whole lot of control, far more than the experts want you believing you have, but you do.

And one hell of a life-changing fact it is. Eighty-five percent of what you do every day affects more than your childhood ever could.

At 260 pounds, I had a pretty slick lineup of reasons why I was so fat. I had them all (including one hell of a childhood), except for the absolutely ridiculous thick-blood thing, which, for the ridiculous record, I've heard more than once.

I had two ten-pound babies a year apart. Talk about physical changes? You bet my body changed after housing two lives, no question about it. For a couple of years two babies in two years was one of my "top five" reasons for being so fat. Until one day the checkout lady at the supermarket asked me when the next baby was due. I wasn't pregnant. My "baby" was well over a year old and he was in my arms, not floating in amniotic fluid inside of me. Honest (I had to be), what was hanging from my stomach was not a baby, it was fat. Nursing two babies, running around after a one- and a two-year-old while the marriage was blowing sky-high, tired anyone. You want tired? Sure, I was adding a little weight, but who wouldn't, after all . . .

So, what to do. I went to my doctor. My OB, for no other reason than I didn't know where else to go . . . who's the specialist for exhaustion? To highlight the significance of my little visit to the doctor that day, let me give you a bit of her-story about where I was during this particular point in my life. Think avalanche. An enormous amount of snow on top of a mountain. Instantly and without warning, a tidal wave of snow breaks thundering down the mountain, burying everything alive in its path. A little too high drama? some may say. Not at all. Every woman reading this who is on her way up the scales and out of her life understands exactly what I'm talking about.

I'd just started another eight-hundred-calorie-day diet, the husband and I were attempting another reconciliation, and I was sitting in my doctor's office crying. Sobbing in public was becoming a normal thing in whoever's life this was that I was living. My visit with the expert that day included:

no mention of the weight I was steadily gaining

no mention of the crappy food I was eating to gain that weight

no suggestion of exercise

No mention of lean muscle mass

No connection to my lifestyle and the unexplainable exhaustion that my life had become . . .

No connection to anything, as a matter of fact. I did get a prescription. That was way before the pharmaceutical boys were the stars of commercial television. Political? I think so; I'm talking 1984. The year, literally, and what has turned into a true story. Meantime, what I got that day from the doctor was a prescription for . . . lithium, fifteen years before the current bipolar craze or the chic of depression. This was back in the day when handing out lithium was serious business, and lithium is what the doctor gave me that day, along with a finger-pointed warning that I needed to calm down as he yelled down the hall to his secretary to schedule an appointment for a thyroid test.

Depression and a possible thyroid problem. Jesus, there's hopeful.

I've heard every "I can't lose this weight" reason under the sun and my response to every one of them is: *get fit*.

No shit, your knee is bad, you've got 150 pounds sitting on top of it; burn a little fat, build some muscular strength, at the very least it'll get much, much better, if not . . . heal. *Heal?* Who, you healing yourself? There's something that pisses the "healers" off.

Well, the fact is: there isn't an affliction in the world that won't be helped by wellness, and most will heal (except, of course, thick blood). Out of the hundreds of reasons I've been given for overfat and unfit, "thick blood" and "addicted to food" are two of my favorites. Thick blood because it's so ridiculous, and addicted to food because . . . no, you are not. That's an insult to junkies, and if you've ever been one, you know what I'm talking about. Heroin is addictive, brownies are not. Imbalanced is what you are if you are eating the shit they are selling you, but addicted you are not. On their sugar roller coaster is where you are, but addicted you are not. Being poisoned, yes, but . . . not addicted.

Truth is, you don't have a thing wrong with you; you, like the other 98 percent of the overfat, unfit population, have simply eaten way too much fat and haven't moved in years, and so that fat is stored. Overfat and unfit may have caused a hundred other problems, 85 percent of all disease being directly connected to lifestyle, but honestly, the way you got fat was/is simple, and the way you are going to get lean is simple, too.

It's time you get honest. Honest about a whole lot of things in your daily life, certainly about the fat that's hanging from all over your body. Honestly, you did it to yourself. You did, like I did. My ex-husband may have been, and is still, an ass, but he wasn't around at 3 a.m. to get me the cake. He was out screwing his girlfriend. I was at home with the kids and eating. It was me who ate the fat to get fat, and it was me who didn't move, and so the fat stored and stored, and it was me who didn't burn it off. The good news is that you did overfat and unfit to yourself, and so you can undo it.

Honestly, you know losing weight isn't complicated, and honestly, you've been steered, for years, toward the promise of the quick fix. Billion-dollar industries can't survive without the nonthinking consumers it takes to keep them in business. And women, the primary victims of quite a few massive industries, are the consumer market holding these boys up high. It's been said, far better than I could ever say it, you cannot be a victim unless . . . ? You've got to lay down to let 'em roll over you. My version of what others have said brilliantly.

Eat, breathe, move, and . . . think because X-changing nonthinking for thinking clears up most of the confusion instantly, and is one of the biggest life-changing things you'll ever do. You clearing up the confusion, by being conscious and honest, makes getting on with the work of burning fat, building strength and energy, and restoring your life a whole lot easier. All the charts, graphs, or scare tactics in the world don't make a difference, and they haven't. The truth must be told and you've got to get conscious and honest about the actions in your daily life that have nothing to with your intentions.

heart disease

arthritis

diabetes

stroke

obesity

cancers

high blood pressure

Honestly, any of it your intention? Of course not, but . . . ? Therein lies the confusion and the daily beating you've been giving yourself for how many years? You know you shouldn't but you do, and when you do you know you shouldn't . . . well, all that is quite simply about to change.

Obviously, there is nothing large and in charge about being overfat and unfit, a statement that creates a tidal wave of response . . . always the resistance. You can't imagine (I can barely imagine it myself) how much hatred is directed at me from the large-and-in-charge feminists. I'm the only person, in the thirty-year history of a particular women's festival, to be boycotted. Festivals that are about nothing but freedom for women. All women except fitness experts? Oh, the stories, the message boards, the chat rooms. In all the years I've publicly had an opinion, I've never seen anything like "the right to fat" feminists demanding body-image respect . . . and my death.

A whole lot of my sisters have no idea that being hugely fat is not a sign of power. Or that what I've been talking about for years—wellness—has nothing to do with looking like the Barbie image (they continually accuse me of upholding) that was designed for women by men. I look like Barbie (on crack) because I like it. It's my choice, and quite deliberate. The fact is, everything I'm saying, whether they like it or not, applies to "every-body," especially feminists. They'd slay me with their labryses before they'll admit it, but my sisters in the women's studies programs are as lobotomized as the mother of five living in the middle of nowhere, cooking up "helpful hamburger things" for the hubby's dinner. The politics of food . . . are you kidding? The fact is, whether you ever use a razor or not (you should have seen me, in broad daylight, shaving every part of my glistening, size-two body in the outdoor festival shower—and I did), or you've never put makeup, that poisoned greasepaint on your face, food is still political. As is wellness.

As is oxygen. Very political. But they won't talk about it because they hate the feminist who is talking about it . . . me. It's stunning but true. Large and in charge—no, you are not; what you are is "killing yourself for the man." Patriarchy doesn't have to do much of anything when women start screaming that overfat and unfit is freedom. The overfat and unfit feminists are doing it for them. Overfat and unfit is patriarchal suicide, ladies, and there is nothing well or okay about it. Large and in charge—no; simply large and metastasizing a deadly message. Nobody can do it better than women, and that includes viciousness. Still, the fact is, starvation and obesity, both food "issues," one the lack of, the other gluttony. Both deadly, done.

I recently picked up an updated copy of the old trail-blazing book *Our Bodies, Ourselves*. Talk about a trip down memory lane and a chance to get reacquainted with the basics of self pelvic exams! There I was in the aisles of the megabookstore/coffeehouse/student lounge flipping through the pages, horrified. Every illustration was of unhealthy, unwell women! What the hell? Anorexic or hugely fat, mainstream or feminists' images . . . both deadly images for women. Fat clogs and kills. The only choices connected to overfat and unfit are a whole bunch of very bad lifestyle choices, choices made daily, and for years.

Honestly, if you'd like to change the way you look and feel, you can. Being honest about one fact changes much. Eighty-five percent of all disease can be directly attributed to lifestyle. All it takes is one very powerful moment if you choose to change yours . . . or you can keep eating the steak and cake and proclaiming self-empowerment. Your choice.

Honestly, if it's you who did it, it's you who can redo it; that's the good news. Just before you do, though, there's one thing that must be discussed: your behavior; your behavior, little lady.

ten

Behavior

Behavior. Another ingredient in the mix that keeps you cemented into doing nothing about this weight problem of yours is your behavior. All the things you do, and why. Heavy duty, deeply connected to your inner child, and way too big a subject to tackle without a degreed person ready to do trauma intervention, right? Wrong. The big scary behavioral breakdown that they've got you convinced has to happen before you lose weight is ridiculous. Behavior modification—yeah, that's worked. Like there's any such thing; it's all just another well-planned snag in your movement forward, and it's a big one because we all have a story. Please, I can tell you stories that would traumatize you from a distance . . . which sounds like a combo: bad Disney theme/country-western-song.

Every one of us has a million reasons why our behaviors are what they are, especially when it comes to the high-fat living we've been doing. You can be fat and talented, fat and have a terrific personality, fat and sew your own clothes . . . you can be fat and a whole lot of things, but you can't be fat and healthy because overfat is unhealthy. Fat kills. Fat creates thousands of other problems that dramatically affect your life daily . . . fat and healthy do not exist in the same body.

If working through all the emotional stuff that some people want you to believe is a prerequisite to losing weight were necessary, I would be five hundred pounds right now. It isn't. Tilting the scales at 250 plus, I could have cared less about self love, toxic waste, animal rights, the planet Earth, or much else, for that matter. I didn't have the energy or strength to get through a day without feeling like I was going to drop dead by the end of it. Care about endangered species when the "aliens" of birth, divorce, isolation, loads of high-fat foods, and no movement had taken over my life, why? I was too tired and not very interested at all in anything other than looking and feeling better. Screw carbon emissions and polar caps melting, why would you think of asking me to save anything when I was busy trying to save myself. Weight loss and world peace . . . I'm getting there.

The truth, is nobody is functional. I've never met a set of parents from our generation who didn't blow it sky-high. Just look at us, all adult children of something. Where would the recovery industries be without our parents' bad parenting? Who hasn't been addicted to something, an enabler of someone, codependent to the nines, or getting their minds messed up by gender, racial, and religious stereotypes? Did I mention I was raised in a Dominican Catholic convent? You can't get much more screwed up than that, and I'm lean, strong, and healthy . . .

Some big closet doors have been blown wide open, the silence is lessening (society being only as sick as its silence), especially now via space, but you sorting at anthing from your past has nothing to do with you losing weight. Get some oxygen while you are sorting it all out, or spending years never getting it sorted out—either way, get some oxygen. Chat with your therapist while you build some lean muscle mass. Spend hours talking about why, while you are eating real food and burning fat. Oy, the resistance when any or all that is even suggested! Why the arguments? Consider nothing but the basics; what you:

A. Can do; and
B. Don't need an expert *to* do

Honestly, who cares that your mother was _____ (fill in the blank)—so was mine. Absent father, much of the time (redundant). Okay. Addicted to . . . yes. Enabler . . . let's talk about my second marriage, shall we (so rhetorical a question). Don't lift a finger, I'll do all the work. Something I still haven't figured out at all, The only difference is, just recently I didn't get married and it wasn't a he.

If you are talking about burning fat, increasing strength and energy, and regaining your body and your brain, you don't have to dig through your childhood or anything else to do just that. All you have to do, and you can (I don't say that as a lifestyle-changing cheerleader; I mean it literally), is add basic life-very-styling biochemics to your daily life. The biochemics of the human body; Dr. Dr. . . . why the resistance? If you must make a connection beyond the eat, breathe, move, and think of it all, why not make a much more prevalent and real connection than trauma. Let's spend a second on just one of the creators of the lifestyle affecting squillions of people. One of the most powerful missiles used to deliver the megablasts against thinking consumers is television.

Something far more influential, when it comes to your life and its lack of style, than your toilet training is the tele. Drone to the fridge every time you are told/sold some rich, high-fat snacky thing. Arms raised, zombie to the ice cream night after night. Late-night eating disorder, or multimillion-dollar advertising campaigns that work? No need to wait for that scientific study to come out, I'm simply suggesting consideration of the possibility that you have been affected/infected. Consider it every time you are about to take the flog from the wall (in your dungeon?) and start flogging.

Fact: You don't have a willpower problem or any problem when it comes to knowing what needs to change in your life. There are many influences that heavily influence beyond your screwed-up family. The choices you make every day affect everything and are directly connected to overfat and unfit. Honestly, the last however many years you've been living as an adult have more to do with everything than most "healers" will ever admit. How you live every day very soon outweighs (pardon the pun) the first eighteen years of your life. At what point do the choices you've been making for years start to matter as much as, if not more than, the trauma? The answer, if you are in therapy, is never . . . which is only one of the reasons why people are in therapy forever. It seems to me that if it worked, it would.

Getting back to basics, one very obvious thing you can do to change one hell of a big lifestyle habit is turn the TV off. Once in a while, more often than not, or forever. Choice . . . it's all about choice, ladies. Start by turning the "autopilot" off; change the background noise in your daily life. Don't automatically turn the thing on every morning or every night. Remember, remind, and redo your television habit: one minute before you automatically turn on the nightly news (nothing new about any of it), which turns into the first sitcom, which turns into the first hour of four, five, six hours of being programmed . . . stop, and do something else. TV doesn't help you build a high-quality life; it's designed to reduce you in every way imaginable, except when it comes to your weight. The truth is, national cookie companies have been making a lot of your life choices for you, with one hell of a powerful penetrator, your TV, which does affect your behavior. Advertising, glamorizing, and normalizing a lifestyle that isn't working for millions is real and, at the very least, must be considered in the state-of-the-nation weight-loss discussions, but never is.

A whole lot more is affecting your behavior than your lack of control. *Behavior,* the meaning of the word explains much.

Behavior: how you act, function, or react in a particular way.

Your choosing not to fall into the bottomless, vague, confusing, complicated, fear-filled pit of every behavioral issue of the past is your answer to more than you can imagine. Quite simply, *behavior* means how you choose to act. And, like calories, not all actions are the same. You, consciously and honestly; choosing how you act changes everything, and has everything to do with weight loss. What affects you much more than your past is your present . . . your present choices, that is.

Behavior = your actions

Action, reaction . . . ?

RE, two letters that changed my thinking back in the day. A very different *re* than the *re* in front of remind, remember, and redo. Nothing new about this *re*, nothing life changing. *Re,* as in the same-old same old. *Re*action. Over and over again, the same *re*sponse. Over and over again, *re*turning to lifestyle habits that don't work in your life. This *re* is the definition of insanity, same thing over and over again and . . . ?

I've got a life-changing formula for you, one that changed my life forever and one that clears up every bit of confusion about you and your behavior.

Action plus repetition = behavior

And it is. No matter what your childhood was like, action plus repetition equals behavior, period. If you'd like another mathematical way of looking at it, try multiplication.

Action times repetition equals behavior; it's true. If it's fat you want to burn and strength and energy you want to increase, sorting through the million things connected to whom you happen to have been born to may not be the only thing you spend your energy, time, and money on. Why not include something as obvious as your daily actions?

At what point is your life your life? The answer is, every day, every choice, cellularly and literally. Action plus repetition equals behavior, and so that behavior eventually becomes your life. Your high-quality, lean, strong, healthy life, or the way you look and feel right now. The design of your life: Fat or fit? Weak or strong? Energized or exhausted? Your body, strong, glowing, comfortable, fitted, oxygenated, or . . . ? Your life is all about the actions you choose to take, or not. Behaviors you've chosen and the behaviors that have been chosen for you—either way you can change them. You've just got to know which action to choose:

.

Reactive or

Proactive

Re as in the same-old same old or *pro* as in professional. You, the professional in your own life . . . now, there's a concept. You at the top of the list of professionals you consult . . . there it is.

Reacting was all over my 260-pound lifestyle. Every time I had a conversation with _____ (fill in that blank) . . . reaction. A night of television . . . reaction. Every time I saw certain family members . . . reaction. Exhausted, raising two babies alone, reaction, reaction, reaction. Two damn letters, *RE,* held the answer to the question that was stalking my brain every day. How can I lose this weight? The lightning bolt that shocked the hell out of me was in the *re.* I'm calling that lifestyle spoken word art which really pisses the spoken word artists off.

If you are reacting to:

the husband

your boss

the kids

the person three cubicles down . . .

Everything, anything . . . If you're reacting to any of these, then it's time you made one hell of a behavior-changing connection. If basic eat, breathe, move, and think behaviors need to change in your life, then reacting has got to go. Because none of it's going anywhere any-time soon . . . until it does.

Do you see the day coming when you don't have to work? I don't know about you, but I'm still working my very lean butt off. It's me who's raising the kids, getting the food bought and cooked, working inside and outside the house, and I don't expect any of that to change any-time soon. Life in all its glory and with its millions of not-so-glorious moments goes on, and you have to change your lifestyle while it does.

The people who had kids and still exercised . . . I never stopped thinking about them once I started thinking. The lean people with idiot ex-husbands stalked me because an indisputable fact was/is that they looked very different from me. I lost my weight by losing the loser thinking that somebody or something was going to magically change my body because I wasn't capable of making the changes I needed to make. Being conscious and honest in the obvious truth.

Fact: If I was going to continue reacting by eating a ton of fat every time _____ (fill in that blank) did some-thing stupid, it didn't take much to figure out I was in some kind of trouble. Same thing applies to extended family; it's not as if reacting to them is going to make them stop being your family anymore, so until they stop being family you have to put up with them. What does that mean to everyone who has family members who annoy the hell out off them? That they're doomed to be fat until everyone in their bloodline gets functional? Same thing applies to . . . everything. Overworked and underpaid . . . that's going to change soon? It hasn't. Not under the current world systems, not if you are a woman.

Women own less than 1 percent of the world's wealth and women do 89 percent of the work that keeps the systems up, running, and enormously profitable, but not for the women. Slavery? How much clearly defined does it need to be. Stress? Yes, there is more stress in this world than most people can handle, but if I hear stress offered as a reason for obesity one more time . . . really. When I was 260 pounds, roaming the house, worried sick, polishing off the pint of ice cream sandwiched between cookies, I was stressed. And just the other night I was roaming the house, worried, and eating everything in sight. I was roaming. I was worried. I was eating ice cream. Not cookies, though, because there weren't any left. With two sons over six feet tall and a growing ten-year-old boy in the house, food may as well be hooked up to an IV and mainlined.

Back in the day, I didn't have enough money to make ends meet, and being hugely fat didn't make being broke any easier. I'm still roaming and worried—just leaner, stronger, and healthier as I roam and worry, which makes roaming and worrying much, much easier.

The difference? I didn't wake in the morning after my binge with more fat on my body, feeling lousy (about myself and biochemically), suffering from refined-white-sugar poisoning. I still eat when I'm sad, worried, or mad. I never learned to modify anything that's obvious, and look at me. I still worry; there's plenty to worry about, so what's changed? Two major things that any human body can change.

what I ate while I roamed

and what I do the morning after worrying and roaming

Increasing the quality of the ice cream I was wolfing down (once a wolfer always a wolfer) and sweating blood the next day. What does it take to increase the quality of ice cream? Nothing.

It's not as if anyone is pretending there is a lot of nutritional value in ice cream, and chances are you will probably eat ice cream during your lifetime, so the question is: "Does it have to be the worst crap on earth?"

the highest fat

most chemicals

dairy

loaded with refined white sugar

No. I changed my lifestyle without working most of my "issues" out. I'm telling you the "eater" didn't figure out how to be a noneater. I just didn't eat a pint of shit. The "undisciplined" person didn't become disciplined. The immature can't-handle-her-emotions person didn't grow up, not an inch. None of that happened, but behaviors did change. I simply learned to get intentional, honest, and proactive in two things that will never, ever change in my life: eating higher-quality foods and moving.

Fact: Honestly, my 260-pound lifestyle choices didn't help my life one bit. Eating a ton of refined white sugar only added to the mess that was my life. Catatonic and poisoned, that works! If you don't think X-ing out (or taking in a ton less) refined white sugar is one of the biggest life-very-styling changes you'll ever make, it's time to start reading something other than the propaganda the refined white boys hand out, because it is.

Honestly: Yes, it was very difficult being 260 pounds and in the middle of a divorce. Making myself sick from my own lifestyle choices did nothing but make it all much worse. I had no idea there would be a couple of bestselling books in the future. Are you out of your mind? It wasn't even a consideration in the middle of those hot summer days in Garland, Texas, just after the fallout of my life. All I knew was that I was going to be waking up in the middle of the night for years to come because one of the kids always had:

chickenpox

allergies

nightmares

a tooth coming through

Fact: There were a few things I could do that would make a huge difference in my life, starting with not getting fatter. Honestly, it wasn't such a big deal to go for a walk no matter how unmotivated I was. And the difference it made in my daily life was indisputable. You can't imagine how enlightened I felt even entertaining the idea that perhaps I could do something other than increase my waistline. When I started making the very real connection between reaction and proaction, I felt like Gandhi. Every time I made the enlightened choice to be *pro*active rather than *re*active I stepped into the light.

Old lifestyle habit . . . reaction.

He didn't show up to visit the kids, again . . . reaction.

New lifestyle habit . . . proactive.

"Okay, he's an idiot, but he's not here right now. Forget about him, think about you." Proactive.

I did it just the other day with a her; same thing. She's an idiot, but she's not here right now . . . you are . . . so how are you going to respond to your life? The exact wording of that answer went through my brain just days ago. Back in the day, every time I made proactive choices in my own life, I knew I was onto something. I didn't have a clue what it was at the time, but I knew it was the white light at the end of the overfat tunnel, so

I hung on for dear life. The action I focused on was getting off *him,* metaphorically speaking of course. Again, he wasn't around to get on . . . and I was getting on with myself.

It wouldn't surprise me if this is news to you, because it was news to me. The art of living is literal. Living, from now on, is reduced to the basic must-haves: oxygen, food, strength, energy . . . a little something something to physically get you through a bloody day. I had to learn how to practice the art of living my life. I had to do the practice (literal) of going from autopilot, bad, life-not-so-styling choices to making intentional, honest, proactive choices, creating new behaviors because that's the way to create new behaviors . . . by creating them. Getting conscious and honest about me and my reactions to all the things around me that were sucking the life out of me is what changed my body and my life forever. It is exactly what will change yours, because a fact of life is, there will be moments in your life of exhilarating joy and moments of crippling pain; all of it exists until none of it does. It's called living. Let's hope that it isn't going to end soon, and you have a much better chance of that not happening if you don't live the all-American lifestyle.

As you progress (*pro*—there's that prefix again) in your new-styling life, connecting some of the really big dots, you will have the protection you need against the old reactions of the past. The *pro*logue of your new life will be written. She's off on a *pro*-prefix tangent, and why not? Just look at the meaning of those three little letters.

Pro. The prefix means: in front of.

Exactly what I've been saying. Instead of the old, branded-into-your-brain, glamorized, socialized, justified fat living reactions you've been living in for too many years, you are going to X-change them for . . . Slap me upside the head if that isn't the exact same thing as X-changing what doesn't work for what does? It's a beautiful thing, this X-changing-reactive-for-proactive thing. I see it every day in the lives of women. Women who used to be overwhelmed, overfat, unfit, and totally and absolutely confused about the most basic (lifestyle) things, and are not anymore. Once you know you don't have to give the kids up for adoption to get as lean, strong, and healthy as you want to get, everything changes—certainly the way you look and feel. You simply have to change behaviors that are not getting you the end results you want in your life, which is completely possible to accomplish. You are still going to be going to work every day; you just won't be getting fatter and fatter. You'll still be the same person you were last week, the person with:

no control

no choice

no idea

no motivation

Just like I'm the same person, only leaner, stronger, and healthier, and perhaps grown a tad. Now when I hear myself say to a lover, "Don't worry, I'll take care of it . . ."

I run. Recently I established new standards for loving someone. They have to:

have a job

be kind and

be able to function

I'm growing all the time, no black marks in my mental-health record recently. I don't mind if you've acted insane in your life, or if you've even been committed once or twice, but something I had to make very clear recently to someone I loved greatly is that if you don't manage your own biochemics once you know what the problem is, you'll *stay* locked up, because I'm not getting you out again and again and again. Matured, I have. Same person, different actions. One life-changing action at a time.

The politics of you changing your own behaviors are obvious. How many experts are going to fall off the face of this earth when millions of women make the connections to all the things they can do that absolutely affect how they look and feel. The politics of weight loss are clear:

The primary victims of the diet industry are women.

The most powerful consumer market in many industries is women.

The consumer market getting the megablasts in the war against an educated consumer is women.

Exactly the reason I speak with, about, and to women. Women are the power even if they have no idea (yet) that they have such power.

World Peace 101, the beginning. At this point in the save-the-earth game, the only hope we have is women. Mothers rising. And if you think I'm talking about women (continually) explaining anything to the boys running our world into the ground, you are dead wrong. I didn't say ask or explain anything. I'm talking about mothers rising and taking back the neighborhood. Mothers rising in fury. Mothers rising and making sure the badly behaved boys aren't allowed to play in the playground with the properly behaved kids anymore . . . mothers rising. This is impossible to do when you are poor; then the price of motherhood is real: too tired, toxic, overfat, and unfit to stand, let alone get through a day.

Target marketing, ladies, and you are heavily targeted. Listen to the language—listen, because it's real. When every woman chooses to increase the quality of her life by increasing the quality of the foods she puts into her body, the ripple effects of that one act alone are stunning: farming, fossil fuel, indigenous everything, massive manufacturing, soil, water, air, poisons, pesticides, pollutants . . . it's global, without a doubt.

You doing something as simple and vital as oxygenating your blood affects/effects everything. Women are the best networkers and connectors on the planet. What used to be called gossip is now called spreading the word. And as I said years ago, the most dangerous animal on earth is . . . ? A pissed-off mother. I speak with women because when a woman gets well, her friends, her community, and eventually the world gets well. One of the most exciting things this window of opportunity called the internet is causing to happen is that women are spreading the word about:

vaccines

autism

ADHD

Ritalin

menopause

obesity

unnecessarily surgical _____ (fill in the blank)

molestation

rape . . . no need for two words to describe the same thing . . .

Mothers against . . . it's about damn time.

There is nothing radical about the fact that women rising will change everything. Have a look, what you'll always see is the multiplication of thousands of problems and the creation of mass confusion. In the meantime, why not start doing the basic biochemics of every human's body? Not to mention—go ahead, twist my arm—the brain activation that goes along with body activation.

Which also means the creativity, sexuality, and inspiration of millions of women will be activated. That's exactly what happens when a body comes back to life . . . it all does. Green being the color these days, what the hell else would the activists want but more activated activists?

Green

The green movement is a movement that makes the hair on the back of my neck stand up because the Politics of Stupid is all over this particular current craze. Oy, the glorification of the White Man, the rich political white man. Don't ever say Nobel Peace Prize to me again because it's lost all meaning, not that it ever had much meaning to women—just look at the ratio. The current leaders of the green movement are the same white men who worked in the administrations that have:

> been doing deals with oil boys for years
>
> passing laws that serve their lobbies for years
>
> jailing the Green Peace boys for years
>
> shutting down every activist for the last sixty years, for God's sake! It's obscene. It makes me want to go back into exile.

White men admitting the world is melting does not a hero make . . . like it's news to hear this? They've known, their administrations knew, and it goes back quite a few administrations, folks, please. I've known for thirty bloody years about global warming. If they'd done something years ago, perhaps there could have been a chance in hell, but not anymore.

Fact: Global warming is not new. In less than one hundred years—years that chronicle the history of the death of a planet (man wins the award for this destruction, bravo) industrialized man has destroyed our world, and it isn't something that is *being* done . . . it *has* been done. Glorifying white men who make movies about our earth melting is obscene, as is the lie that they have solutions to change things for the better. The men who created the problem in the first place cannot solve it. The earth will mutate . . . she does, and you'd better mutate also if you want to survive. Again, enter fitness. Yes, I said fitness just after "mutate if you want to survive," because it applies, never more so than now, when epidemic diseases are real.

How many times can you gasp in horror when you hear of a twenty-eight-year-old, a thirty-three-year-old, with cancer. How many times are you going to pretend it's a horrifying, isolated, sad incident . . . because it's not. Cancers are epidemic, "getting far more aggressive," and are being seen in younger and younger people. What I witnessed just a couple of months ago is real. The details (unfortunately for the victims) don't matter. I got a phone call, a friend's husband had a really bad backache, so they took him to the hospital on a Thursday night. Four weeks later, he's dead. Cancer everywhere. I've heard the same story twice this summer. The names of the victims change, but the story doesn't, and it's not going to. There are real consequences to:

breathing polluted air

drinking polluted water

eating processed, poisoned food grown in demineralized, chemical-soaked soil, and we are

Then, along comes the white man (run if you have any dignity left) with ten tips on how to save the planet! Never the truth, always the detour. Meantime, the fact is . . .

Fact: Man has "ruled" for over five thousand years. They've had their run, and they have buggered it up completely and absolutely. No question about it.

The solution is women, and I'm not talking about a women's movement . . . there is none. There's not even a good bowel movement in this country right now, let alone a woman's movement. The "movement" is far too busy considering everybody and everything. The movement has become the generic good wife: make sure you include every gender, trauma, physical handicap . . . God knows you don't want to offend. Anyone who's ever tried to get anything done with a panel of women knows that it's impossible. The only way this world is going to have a chance in hell to survive is when every woman, each woman, makes the vitally important connection between her body and her brain. Wellness and world peace—the connection I'm making more strongly by the second. When you understand the politics behind biological suicide, the bio-chemical warfare being waged against you and your children, we have a chance for change. Until then, we're screwed.

Can you imagine how popular I am in the movements—the feminist and green ones—but what I'm saying is the truth. What better time and reason to talk about it—our world as we know it is melting. How many species disappearing by the second do you need? Humans are . . . ? A species. If the polar bears can disappear, so can you, honey. Think, think, think about it.

If it's world peace you'd like to talk about, let's. The only way it's gonna happen is when patriarchy ends. Male governed . . . owned . . . profited from (redundant) . . . translated . . . enforced must end. What I'm suggesting is a complete takeover of the planet. I didn't say "equal" or "share," I said "take (not ask to take) over." Women taking over the world, that's what I'm talking about, and that's the only way there is ever going to be world peace.

Weight loss is a given when you change the lifestyle that makes you fat, but weight loss has never been my primary motivation. It's your brain I've always been interested in.

You rising from the living death that millions of women are barely surviving in daily is the solution to more than most people could ever imagine possible. You joining the mothers who are done with the same-old same old, and there are plenty of us. The mothers who are no longer asking politely if you'd stop raping our babies and us. Mothers who live daily as if the air they breathe also belongs to them. Mothers living as if the earth they live on was theirs. Mother's living daily as if the choices they make *affect,* because they do. And before we get to the takeover of the world (it'll lead there organically), you being able to design and implement something as simple as how the hell you choose to look and feel every day is clearly the place to start. The most revolutionary thing any woman can do is to take charge of her internal wellness. Which is only one of the things I say that my sisters hate, but it's true. Your responsibility in all this? Exactly what we need to discuss. The last word of your life-changing program is *responsibility,* little lady.

eleven

Responsibility

Responsibility, the very thing we need to talk about in order for you to completely understand how your life is going to change, and it's not what you think. Your responsibility to you, your body, and the world starts with you wiping out everything you ever thought was responsible. As with everything else, you've only been given a one-dimensional version of responsibility.

Before consulting *Webster's,* here's my new and much-improved definition of the word *responsibility,* a more literal definition. Look at the word.

Responsibility: your response to your ability.

Ta-da! Your response to your ability to . . . ? You increasing your response to your ability. Think about that totally different definition of a word that, up until now, hasn't done you a bit of good. Your ability to . . . let's talk about a blank that needs to be filled in. If anything is going to change in your life, definitely your body, you are going to have to increase your response to your ability to do a few things. This is a big statement, not because it's difficult to do . . . it's a big statement because it changes everything. You increasing your response to your ability is the (real) weight-loss guarantee. One hell of a lifestyle X-change that (again and again and again) is never mentioned in the endless weight-loss discussions, unless, as always, they are talking about your complete lack of ability. No weight-loss infomercial producer will touch the word *responsibility* with a ten-foot pole unless you are willing to believe that the ten-foot pole is really a magic weight-loss wand. If any variation of the word *responsibility* is going to be a part of a weight-loss seminar or workshop, you run the risk of being uninvited before the party ever begins.

Apparently, you can't stomach the suggestion. It's not a word you are interested in, it's:

too harsh

too much to ask

too overwhelming

too blatant

too difficult

not glamorous enough

I've been told (over and over again) that suggesting you take responsibility for how you live takes away from the perceived value of a weight-loss program. It's too truthful and you are not interested in the truth. I'd be glad to give you the names and numbers of the boys who've said to me, "Give 'em a chart, give 'em a graph, make it look programmatic. The truth will take the glamour out of it." Exactly what I've been told will happen if the R-word is uttered. Perhaps now you can see why I'm not invited to many of my motivational-speaker peers' motivational things. Being the team player that I'm not, and given what's liable to come out of my mouth, inviting me is far too much of a risk. They can't afford (literally) to have me join them because I won't go along with "the program." "What program?" The program of making people believe that there *is* some program . . . because there isn't.

Guru status is not hard to get. I have it. It's not a word I ever use—*guru*—but it is a word that is used often to describe people like me. "Fitness guru." The fact is, I'm a housewife who figured something (a few things) out and started talking to other women. I'm not allowed on the mountaintop or in the pulpit because I have a vagina. As far as I'm concerned, mountaintop or pulput, it's the same thing with different headdresses, and neither works for me. What does work for me is intuitive wisdom and common sense, and when it comes to you increasing your response to your ability to do everything you want to do, all you need is common bloody sense.

Webster's says responsibility means:

*The state of being responsible. Called upon to answer
for one's acts or decisions. Accountable for important
duties. Able to fulfill one's own obligations. Trustworthy. Reliable.*

Accountable for your acts and decisions, yes. Very rea-
sonable when you think about it. Able to fulfill your own
obligations to . . . ? Yep, guess who? You. Trustworthy
and reliable; exactly what you are to half the world, to everyone except . . . ? It would be rude of me to push this
point because it's as obvious as daylight.

Change a choice, change your life. Change your
choices, consciously, honestly, proactively, and you will
change the way your body looks and feels. You increasing
your response to your ability is the cell of change. Any
and all change, but when it comes to this "weight issue" of
yours, it's the be all and the end all. You getting intentional and honest about your life and it's style, proactive
in your behaviors (X-changing one high-fat, inactive lifestyle habit at a time), all the while increasing your response to your ability, and it's done.

I heard something years ago that changed my thinking forever. "The only way to change bad habits is to re-
place them with better ones." Exactly what you are going
to do with your whole life. One high-fat, processed-to-
death food choice at a time. One inactive-to-active habit
at a time. One bad-lifestyle habit at a time, which is the
only way to change your whole life. The how is now, and
it only takes a minute. Your remind, remember, and redo

moments have a name. A name that haunts me, no matter how hard I've tried to come up with something less ridiculous. The fact is, the moment of change has a name:

The Power of the Pause.

All the power you'll ever need is in a pause. The power of the pause, which in my mind conjures images of Goldie Hawn go-go dancing on *Laugh-In,* which should tell you a lot about my mind. Yes, your program is a one-minute program. All the weight you've ever needed to lose can be lost in one minute. A squillion one minutes for the rest of your life. Because your life is the decisions you make daily. Your life has more to do with what you have eaten, breathed, moved, and thought for the last however many years than it has to do with who you were born to. Your life changes when you change your choices, and from now on, that's a fact of every human body's life, absolutely every human who wants to change her body.

Consider the power of the pause the reading, writing, and 'rithmetic of life changing. The one, two, three of reweaving the new fabric of your daily life. It's simple if you actually do it, which isn't as easy as it sounds, not for me. Stopping for a full minute, sixty seconds, almost killed me. Stopping over for one minute isn't something my genetic structure does naturally. Like meditating . . . it's just not for me. Back in the day, a dear friend of mine went on a ten-day retreat to an ancient monastery and invited me along. I jumped at the chance, me there, sign me up, wipe the schedule clean . . . there are some things in this life that are worth doing no matter what you need to rearrange in order to do them. "Okay, boys, Mommy's going retreating." And then I heard the next thing out of the mouth of my friend. Ten days of silence! she said. Ten days . . . no talking. Not a sound.

Alrighty, mix me a cyanide cocktail and ask me if I'd like a sip . . . because ten days of silence would amount to the same thing. Apparently, my dear friend (who didn't seem to know me at all) forgot that ten days of silence would kill me. I could see the headline: EX-FAT WOMAN IMPLODES IN ANCIENT MONASTERY. "No thank you, have fun healing" was my answer to that invite. But, life changer, be aware, nothing quite so complicated is required of you. Indeed, it's the no-brainer of a lifetime. All you have to do is add three more words to your vocabulary, three simple steps to your life. Just after remember, remind, and redo comes:

stop

look, and

listen

Stop, which creates the pause which (oh, you bet) creates the space in which you are going to remember, remind, and redo your life. Details be damned, because now details are live, "direct" from me to you, always and forever at www.susanpowteronline.com. Stay with me here and now. Nothing can heal in imbalance. There isn't a healer on the planet who'd disagree with that. Women are more than one half of this world's population and . . . ? Exactly. Political? Without a doubt. Take over? Why not? Asking has done us no good. Domestic violence is at a worldwide, all-time high. Five hundred thousand women were raped in the United States last year alone. Over 65 percent of the poverty-level households in this country are headed by single mothers. Enough said . . . imagine. Women no longer accepting any of it is how, where, and when world peace will happen, and I believe, with every cell of my being, that this can only happen with the practical application of lifestyle changing by—yep, me, Susan Powter.

I'd better send the Nobel Peace Prize givers the correct spelling of my last name, don't you think? Why the hell not? Is anything else working? Have any of the thousands of theories done you a bit of good? No, but this will because you are going to do it. First, you are going to review it with me.

Lifestyle X-change program in review

We agree. You are not the only problem (operative word, *only*) when it comes to this weight issue of yours, correct? Is it fair to say there are other, outside influences—there, that's me being objective.

From now on, when you are ready to pull the whip from the wall, you are going to, at the very least, include:

multibillion-dollar ad campaigns designed to infect

thousands of massive corporations who profit greatly from disease and whose P&Ls depend on the spreading of many diseases

Some of your new, very styling thinking is the truth: the all-American lifestyle, a lifestyle that has been cemented into the brains of millions for well over sixty years (history of the fast-food boys alone, have a look). A lifestyle that is being branded (hot iron to the flesh) into the brains of generations . . . isn't working.

The fact that said lifestyle isn't working for more than just you (you lazy slob) and your family (you bad, bad parent, you) isn't coincidental and you vow to include it in your thinking (from this day forward).

You now know, and will always equally include basic biology every time you are forced to dwell in all the other ologies. Not to mention living with me, but twist my arm.

Lifestyle means what you eat, breathe, move, and think.

Eighty-five percent of all disease can be directly connected to lifestyle.

Obesity is a lifestyle issue.

Change your lifestyle and you solve the problems of overfat and unfit, forever.

And today, the first day of your lifestyle X-change program, you are going to start with two very basic things: move and eat. X-changing two major lifestyle habits. Inactive to active, a massive styling change. Crappy food for whole, nutrient-rich food, which is change on a cellular level.

Oxygen

Today you are going to move in oxygen for thirty minutes or more whether you are inspired to or not, which means you are:

feeding every cell and muscle in your body

activating your metabolic rate

burning fat

building cardio endurance and strength

oxygenating your body and your brain . . .

And you are going to remember and remind yourself of that. Motivation is in the process of doing; once you do, you'll get more and more motivated.

Today, you are going to build what is the most active tissue in every human being's body: lean muscle mass. When you do, you will do just that, build the most active tissue in every human being's body, lean muscle. Fifteen minutes with your thirty minutes in oxygen, and bingo, you've got a forty-five-minute workout routine.

Eat

Today you are going to make higher-quality, whole, real food choices, which means you are:

fueling your body with high-quality fuel

activating your metabolic rate

supplying the gas for the car to run

feeding every cell and muscle in your body

affecting everything from farming to the air you breathe

finally acting like the queen of the aisle that you absolutely are

changing your life, without an expert in sight . . . except you, of course

Today you are going to do three things—two, actually—because moving and breathing are directly connected . . . eat . . . breathe . . . move, and . . . then today you are going to add one more very styling life change.

Today you are going to think. The minute, every minute, for a minute you reach for the old and tired lifestyle habits of the past, you are going to:

stop

look

listen

And:

remember

remind

redo

And change your life.

The politics are obvious. A lifestyle that has been designed, funded, and implemented for everybody who lives in our culture today is killing millions.

American invasion has reached far beyond the world wars (and it is plural; they just have millions of people focused where they want them focused right now) and the American invasion goes far beyond the current administration's mess. Just like global goes way beyond banking. Chemical warfare is literal. No need to focus on sandy deserts far across the world, where law and order is being restored—no, no. The biochemical warfare I see every time I walk down the street is real and can easily be solved by you, which in turn will sure as hell help you make the stand that must be made now. Weight loss and world peace is one of the simplest connections to make. Women are the primary victims of _____ (fill in that blank). Millions of women who are too tired and toxic to do anything about much more than trying to get through a day works brilliantly—but not for the women. If you'd like to see clearly how weight loss and world peace are directly connected, reverse "it." Reverse what you've been told weight loss is. Reverse everything you've ever heard about losing weight and you'll see what it is they don't want you to see.

Weight loss now means wellness. Wellness means oxygen, strength, energy, and your activated body and brain. You knowing that means you have the solution to a massive (pardon the pun) problem facing millions of loving, bright, well-intentioned citizens of this world. Getting back to world balance and world peace is easily spotlighted with one question. A question that gives you the solution for everything.

Are women . . .

50 percent of the world's governments?

Are women

50 percent of the world's religions?

Are women

50 percent of the world's corporations?

Are women

50 percent of the world's educational systems?

Are women

50 percent of the world's sciences?

The most rhetorical of all questions, which begs the question "Why the hell not?" In the meantime, women getting physically lean, strong, healthy, and well would certainly help, wouldn't you say? And "any-body" who wouldn't would be stupid. Wellness, by, Susan Powter.